History of Medicine

It is sobering to realise that as recently as the year in which On the Origin of Species was published, learned opinion was that diseases such as typhus and cholera were spread by a 'miasma', and suggestions that doctors should wash their hands before examining patients were greeted with mockery by the profession. The Cambridge Library Collection reissues milestone publications in the history of Western medicine as well as studies of other medical traditions. Its coverage ranges from Galen on anatomical procedures to Florence Nightingale's common-sense advice to nurses, and includes early research into genetics and mental health, colonial reports on tropical diseases, documents on public health and military medicine, and publications on spa culture and medicinal plants.

Dissertations on Malaria, Contagion and Cholera

When this book was first published in 1832, England was caught in a cholera pandemic that had already claimed hundreds of thousands of lives across Europe. It was commonly held that 'bad air' spread the disease, but theories and remedies varied: one doctor advised the Nottinghamshire public to carry silk cushions filled with myrrh and camphor to strengthen resistance to contagion, while in New York officials suspected that raw vegetables and cold water were the root of the problem. In this fiercely logical treatise, ship's doctor William Aiton cuts through even the most prevalent myths to investigate the pandemic's real causes. Throwing out the theory of bad air, he observes that cholera spreads most quickly in cities with a stagnant water supply and overseas trade. Also addressing the spread of other infectious diseases, his work provides an invaluable insight into the conflicting information available to the general public during pandemics.

Cambridge University Press has long been a pioneer in the reissuing of out-of-print titles from its own backlist, producing digital reprints of books that are still sought after by scholars and students but could not be reprinted economically using traditional technology. The Cambridge Library Collection extends this activity to a wider range of books which are still of importance to researchers and professionals, either for the source material they contain, or as landmarks in the history of their academic discipline.

Drawing from the world-renowned collections in the Cambridge University Library and other partner libraries, and guided by the advice of experts in each subject area, Cambridge University Press is using state-of-the-art scanning machines in its own Printing House to capture the content of each book selected for inclusion. The files are processed to give a consistently clear, crisp image, and the books finished to the high quality standard for which the Press is recognised around the world. The latest print-on-demand technology ensures that the books will remain available indefinitely, and that orders for single or multiple copies can quickly be supplied.

The Cambridge Library Collection brings back to life books of enduring scholarly value (including out-of-copyright works originally issued by other publishers) across a wide range of disciplines in the humanities and social sciences and in science and technology.

Dissertations on Malaria, Contagion and Cholera

Explaining the Principles Which Regulate Endemic, Epidemic, and Contagious Diseases, with a View to Their Prevention

WILLIAM AITON

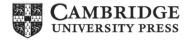
CAMBRIDGE
UNIVERSITY PRESS

CAMBRIDGE UNIVERSITY PRESS

Cambridge, New York, Melbourne, Madrid, Cape Town,
Singapore, São Paolo, Delhi, Mexico City

Published in the United States of America by Cambridge University Press, New York

www.cambridge.org
Information on this title: www.cambridge.org/9781108061414

© in this compilation Cambridge University Press 2013

This edition first published 1832
This digitally printed version 2013

ISBN 978-1-108-06141-4 Paperback

DISSERTATIONS

ON

MALARIA, CONTAGION,

AND

CHOLERA;

EXPLAINING THE PRINCIPLES WHICH REGULATE

ENDEMIC, EPIDEMIC, & CONTAGIOUS DISEASES,

WITH A VIEW TO THEIR PREVENTION:

INTENDED AS

A GUIDE

TO

MAGISTRATES, CLERGYMEN, AND HEADS OF FAMILIES.

By WILLIAM AITON, M.D.

MEMBER OF THE ROYAL COLLEGE OF SURGEONS OF LONDON;
EXTRAORDINARY MEMBER OF THE ROYAL MEDICAL SOCIETY OF EDINBURGH;
AND SURGEON OF THE ROYAL NAVY.

"The means of prevention are more within our power than those of cure."

Sir G. BLANE.

LONDON:

LONGMAN, REES, ORME, BROWN, GREEN, & LONGMAN,
PATERNOSTER ROW.

MDCCCXXXII.

TO

His Most Excellent Majesty

WILLIAM THE FOURTH.

SIRE,

From the benevolent attention of your Majesty
to every department of the Navy, and from your most
gracious condescension to receive any suggestions which tend
to promote the welfare of every class of your Majesty's subjects, sprung my first hope and best encouragement to solicit
the honor of that permission which now enables me to place
the following sheets under the most gracious protection and
distinguished patronage of your Majesty.

I have the honor to be,

With profound respect,

SIRE,

Your Majesty's most obedient,

and most devoted humble Servant,

WILLIAM AITON.

PREFACE.

I HAVE long been of opinion, that a book on the causes of endemic, epidemic, and contagious diseases was much wanted, and that he who should execute the task, even with ordinary care and ability, would deserve well of the public. Our knowledge of endemics and epidemics does not seem to have kept pace with that of other branches of medical science, nor have the investigations into the nature of their causes been always conducted on the same principles. This may be one reason why it has not been equally successful; but, besides this, the extent of the subject, the multiplicity of matters its consideration involves, and the numerous difficulties that beset the path of enquiry almost at every step, must likewise be taken into the account. I am not acquainted with any author who has collected all the principal facts known regarding marsh and morbid poisons into a focus, so as to bring them to bear on the most disputed points, nor any one who has even attempted to explain the different phenomena connected with the rise, progress, and decline of epidemic diseases on scientific principles. Many ancient and modern writers have recorded important facts concerning them, but these have generally been obscured by partial statements, tending to support some favourite theory ; and each succeeding speculation will be found to assume something of the aspect and fashion of the time at which it was first promulgated. Hence, the lights which the occult sciences furnished, no sooner vanished in their native darkness, than a crowd of ærial visions arose, and these were gifted with mechanical or chemical powers, according to the taste of the enquirer. For philosophers to descend at once from the heavenly bodies to earthly concerns, or at least to objects nearer the earth, was undoubtedly a great step gained.

The mathematical physicians who *figured* for some time, were succeeded by the chemists, and these again became acid, alkaline, septic, or antiseptic theorists, according to their own particular views or the progress of chemical science at the time they wrote. All this was natural enough, and even praiseworthy, and had they always adopted the mode of inquiry recommended by Bacon, no fault could have been found either with them or their theories ; but fancy was not to be thus fettered. Accordingly several, even of the most learned of our modern writers, prefer the road of utter darkness to one provided with many lights, and on which many foot-marks may be found to point out the right course.

I have chosen the latter mode of procedure, convinced that it is better to creep along the right path, than to fly on that which is wrong. During the last five and twenty years, I have endeavoured to travel this weary road. I have examined the causes of disease in every climate, and in the different quarters of the world. I have watched them in public and in private life, and in almost every rank and condition of society, and I have carefully examined them in the writings of almost all the best authors, ancient and modern. What use I have made of these advantages is a different question.

In the road of enquiry, I have followed closely the footsteps of those I believed to be the best guides and pioneers, leaving their tract only where they appeared to tread on slippery ground. At the cross-roads I have read the different sign-posts, and tried to profit by every beacon; where even these failed to direct me. I have not scrupled to lay hold of any object that seemed to invite my grasp. On some points which have been long and much disputed, I have thought it best to give the evidence adduced by our best writers. The authorities I have given, will have more weight with the public than any thing derived from my own experience.

Those who have not had opportunities of making themselves acquainted with the history of epidemic diseases, may blame me for laying too little stress on the influence of the atmosphere; but, when it is considered how often mankind have been misled by wrong theories concerning it, and how little statistical medicine has been regarded by many even of our best authors on epidemic diseases, I hope it will be conceded, that I have given to both doctrines a full and fair examination.

There is scarcely a great epidemic, plague, typhus, or yellow fever on record, which was not attributed, at its commencement, chiefly to some known or hidden quality of the atmosphere, while the doctrine of contagion and importation was rejected as a vulgar belief, for the want of what is called direct evidence; every wind that prevailed, and every accidental change of weather which happened at the time, were not only eagerly laid hold of by those who believed they knew more about the matter than their fellow mortals, but were at once held forth by them as the most convincing evidence. The fatal consequences of such vague and conjectural notions were just what might have been expected. Before the real causes of the evil became manifest to all unprejudiced persons, the diseases in most instances gained such ground that all human efforts to stop their progress proved unavailing, and thus the prejudices of the ignorant as to the efficacy of human means of prevention were sure of being strengthened.

The injurious tendency of wrong notions regarding the general atmosphere has not been confined to great epidemics. This heart-reviving fluid has been blamed for many of the evils occurring in private life; thus, the fashionable lady who injures her health and her looks by late hours and crowded assemblies, the pampered profligate who derives his illness from his own dissipation, the bon-vivant who indulges himself into gout, the delicate female starved into a consumption by improper clothing and food, with many more unhappy and unfortunate invalids, have all recourse to the general atmosphere, as affording an easy and ready solution of every pathological difficulty.

Let me, therefore, appeal to the good sense of the public on the subject of cholera, and let me conjure them not to throw away the lessons afforded by past experience. Those who peruse the flimsy productions of the newspaper press on the subject of its atmospheric origin, will not blame me for over-zeal, if they calmly consider the principles on which such theories are founded. 1st. We are told that *undue proportions of the gases composing the atmosphere* are the causes of cholera, though the same quantity of each be found in the air of different countries and at different heights from the earth's surface. 2nd. *Cholera depends upon certain winds;* yet it has often been confined for a time to a single spot of the countries it visited. When it does break out, it does not spread like influenza over a whole community, but is confined at first to one individual, to one room, to one house, to one street, to one town; it then goes to another place to observe a similar mode of procedure. In shifting its residence, it progresses with equal facility contrary to the wind as it does with it, and it continues its ravages in a place during every kind of wind as when there is no wind. 3rd. *It arises from climate and season,* although it breaks out in different places at uncertain periods, and in all climates and seasons alike. Vast tracts of the inhabited parts of the globe have not yet been visited, although they possess the climate and seasons supposed to be favourable to its existence. 4th. *Cholera derives its origin from certain soils;* yet marshy, sandy, and clay soils, in every condition of moisture and dryness, with shingle, rich loam, poor gravel and hard rock, produce it. In other words, places possessing every kind of soil and places having no soil. 5th. *It owes its origin to vegetables;* yet it rages in ships at sea, where men die from the want of

vegetables. 6th. *Certain localities produce it,* although
it marches with seeming indifference in cultivated and
in barren places, over mountainous districts the same
as on level plains, over water as on dry land, and a
great proportion of the civilized world has fallen under
its malign influence. Lastly—*Cholera is guided by
the electric fluid;* yet its rapidity in travelling, never
exceeds that of human intercourse in the countries it
visits. Such is a synopsis of the atmospheric theory
of cholera. To give credence to such a theory, is to
believe in the existence of *something* arising from
nothing, yet a being independent of *everything.* On
the other hand, if cholera be compared with other
contagious epidemics, an account of which I have
given in the following pages—the reader will be the
better able to form a correct notion regarding its
nature and origin.

The matter in the following pages was intended to
form part of a larger work on the Principles of Health,
in which the causes of diseases and their prevention
were to be fully considered ; but, as I thought the part
now published might be useful to the public in the
present crisis, I have chosen to print it in separate
dissertations, rather than delay till the whole was
ready for the press. The part on cholera was written
several weeks ago. With regard to style, I have to
crave indulgence from the public, never having before
written for the press. The manuscript was chiefly
written amidst the noise and bustle of a man-of-war,
whilst I was on service on the Mediterranean Sea, but
from materials previously collected. Here, I regret to
say, I had not access to the works of the authors

quoted, nor much convenience for making the best use of my notes. I have annexed a full table of contents, with a view of directing the student to what I consider to be the best sources for obtaining further information, as also to acknowledge my obligations to the different living authors from whose writings I have extracted much important matter. I have had occasion to differ in opinion from some, whose character for learning and talent, must ever stand high with the profession ; I shall be sorry if my motives for disregarding their authority on some occasions be misconstrued.

Note.—It is necessary to mention that the *cholera*, spoken of at page 25 of the Fifth Dissertation, is the usual form of the disease which is generally acknowledged to be a distemper arising chiefly from high temperature, and not the contagious cholera. I beg to refer those who may wish to see a fuller explanation of the principles which I profess to have followed in the present work, to my concluding remarks at page 212.

ERRATA.

MALARIA ·—Page 47, line 14, *for* common, *read* cannon shot.

CONTAGION:—Page 7, line 7, *for* Sinæpeus, *read* Sinopæus.
             13,   3, *for* than in others, *read* than others.
             20,   12, *for* than to others, *read* than others.
             97, in foot note, *for* fallacious, *read* deceptive.
           124,   9, *for* Satch, *read* Sætch.
         181, line 31, *for* chink, *read* drink.
         188,   17, *for* phlagiston, *read* phlogiston.
         192,   33, *for* a fomites, *read* a fomes.
         199,   32, *for* Magendi, *read* Magendie.
                     for Breschet, *read* Bresslet.

PART II.

DISSERTATIONS ON HEALTH.

NATURAL CAUSES CONTINUED.

MALARIA, AND MARSH MIASMATA.

THE natural state of the two great elements, air and water, is motion. Motion is as essential to the purity of both, as circulation is to the blood and exercise to the human body. In this state air and water are kept from impregnation with foreign matters, both having a power of self-preservation which they do not possess in an equal degree when in a quiescent or stagnant condition. Where water does not gurgle from a fountain, foam in a cascade, or run in a stream, certain saline particles are added to it in order to preserve it from change; but even this would scarcely be sufficient were it not for the perpetual motion and frequent storms which are seen on the face of the troubled ocean. Thus the very means which the great Author of our being employs for the purity of the water of the ocean, have also the effect of preserving the air from corruption. When air and water are in a quiescent state, a third great element, caloric, exerts its powers with greater effect : the water, being partly evaporated, rises into the atmosphere during the day, but in the evening, as the sun has declined in power, this vapour falls again upon the earth in the form of dew, as the air, when condensed by

B

cold, has no longer the power of retaining the same quantity of water. When this vapour descends it does not always fall immediately upon the earth, but is often suspended, in the evenings especially, in the form of fog. The cause of this is, that the earth, retaining a considerable portion of that heat imparted to it during the day, continues to evaporate water for some time after the sun's rays are withdrawn.

The vapours thus exhaled by the earth's heat are no longer capable of rising high into the atmosphere for the reasons already stated, but the ascending vapours meeting the descending, both are for a time suspended near the earth's surface. Something of the same kind happens in the mornings during certain states of atmosphere, till the force of the sun's rays again dissipates the vapours near the earth's surface, and, rarifying the air, thus enables it to retain more moisture.

Fog, then, is merely a visible aggregate of minute drops of water suspended in the atmosphere. The same aggregate which in this situation obtains the name of fog or mist, is called cloud in the higher regions of the atmosphere, but it is concluded, from numerous observations, that the particles of which a cloud consists are always more or less electrified. This is the common effect produced by heat or caloric on water, and we have explained the reason why all exhalations from the earth's surface become generally more dangerous to health in the evenings and mornings.

If the air, during this change, be in a quiescent state, it will very soon become saturated with moisture ; but if it be in motion, the same thing does not happen, because the air, before it becomes saturated, is carried away, and is constantly succeeded by that which is dryer. It is in this way that wind acts in drying moist bodies so much better than stagnant air. The same thing explains why calm weather in certain situations proves injurious to health.

Water during evaporation carries off a proportion of caloric from whatever body it is raised, but this abstraction of caloric, like the process we have just explained, is dependant on the atmosphere, for if it be at the time in a state of rest, much less water will be evaporated, and, of course, less heat be abstracted.

The influence of evaporation in cooling bodies, or, which is the same thing, abstracting caloric from them, has been long known. Wine is cooled by suspending the bottles containing it in bags, and throwing water over them from time to time. The houses in India are kept comparatively cool by evaporation artificially produced. Some fluids may be frozen by the evaporation of other fluids, and death itself may be induced by similar means.

But, besides this influence on the temperature of bodies, evaporation acts an important part in other points of view. Vapour is the cause of clouds, rain, and dew, all of which purify the atmosphere even mechanically, but by promoting vegetation they impregnate the atmosphere in various ways; in particular, odoriferous, volatile, and aromatic substances are separated from herbs and plants, and a due supply of oxygen, or vital air is afforded. Heat, then, is the cause of cold ; difference of temperature in places produces perflation in the air ; and motion of the air will be followed by motion in the water also. Thus the two great elements, air and water, are kept in a healthy condition, partly by the agency of a third—caloric.

Hitherto we have confined our observations to the ordinary operation of the elements on each other. Other effects of the combined operation of air, water, and caloric, must now come into view. These three agents act a principal part in supporting and maintaining animal and vegetable life : but as life is the cause of death, and the end of both animals and plants is made to depend upon their beginning, so the very same agents operate in inducing disease, death, and decay, in all organised matter. This decay, or decomposition of dead organised matter, is known by the general term *putrefaction,* in promoting which, air, moisture, and caloric, are the principal agents. But death and decay of organised matter make

B 2

way for new and vigorous life, nay, are the direct means of a succeeding growth, maturity and death. For the putrefying vegetable becomes the food and nourishment of the living, and this in its turn yields subsistence to the animal kingdom. In short, in the whole circle of the natural world we never witness a single instance of destruction or annihilation.

It is plain, however, that this important process of decay, or putrefaction, must be kept within certain bounds. For, if all animals and vegetables were to live the same length of time, or die at the same age, or if the process of after-decay, or putrefaction, had been regulated exactly by the same laws in all of them, instead of it yeilding nourishment, and giving vigour to living animals and plants, putrefaction must have been the cause of instant death to all living organised matter. Such a degree of corruption would have been inconsistent with life of any kind. Fortunately, however, this danger has been wisely guarded against by Nature.

As the air acts upon the water, the water upon the air, and caloric upon both, by certain fixed and unalterable laws only, so the process of decay in dead organised matter is regulated and restrained within bounds, beyond which it cannot pass.

Perhaps no subject which man is capable of conceiving is more worthy of his admiration and his praise.

It is generally admitted that no substances are capable of putrefaction but such as have been elaborated by the principles of animal and vegetable life. All the agents employed by Nature in the process are perhaps not yet known, but heat, moisture, air, and rest or stagnation, are all essential for this purpose. Certain modifications or degrees of these, according with the different inherent properties of the different animal and vegetable substances opposed to their operation, will undoubtedly decompose dead organised matter, of whatever kind. The mode in which these different agents operate now fall to be explained. All bodies in nature, whether living or dead, are subject to the action of two opposite forces, the natural attraction of their particles on the one hand, and the repulsive power of caloric on the other. So that bodies exist in the solid, liquid, or gaseous state as one or other of these forces prevail. Certain counteracting causes, therefore, operate in retarding putrefaction. Where the attraction subsisting between the particles or component parts of any body is very powerful, of course the repulsive power of caloric will have less effect, and the substances will go slower into putrefaction. On the other hand, when air or water, or their elementary principles happen to possess a stronger attraction for some of the elementary principles of the dead organised matter, than the elements composing them have amongst themselves, the repulsive power of caloric may not be so necessary to promote their separation, in other words, the decomposition. In this way the agency of heat, air, and moisture, in promoting putrefaction, is partly explained.

The effect of rest or stagnation in this process is easily understood, for bodies of different natures not only require to be in close contact for some time before they can act effectually on each other, so as to produce a chemical change, but they must remain sometimes in the due proportions required, otherwise no change in their component parts can take place. When the two agents, air and water, are in motion, the temperature, to say nothing of the arrangement of particles in the dead organised matter, must necessarily undergo perpetual change. Another effect of stagnant water or air falls to be noticed.

The products of putrefaction, in other words the elementary parts of dead organized matter, are not let loose when separated from each other, as some people imagine, to corrupt the air and water.

Under ordinary circumstances these products, whether in a gaseous or other state, soon enter into new combinations, which are hurtful to neither air nor water; both being protected from such change by laws of their own. Those products of putrefaction which cannot find new combinations on the spot where they are separated, are carried by the wind and water to other places more favourable for new formations. In this way the whole may soon be taken up. Where the air and water are in a state of rest however, it may so happen that a greater quantity of the elements of dead organized matter may be disengaged by the process of putrefaction in a place than what can find a new alliance in that particular spot; and these products, not having the advantage of either air or water in a state of motion to convey them to other situations more favourable for this purpose, may thus corrupt both the stagnant air and water in that particular locality to such a degree, as to prove hurtful to animal and even vegetable life.

Heat acts in promoting putrefaction as it does in other instances, by lessening the force of attraction subsisting between the elementary particles of dead organized matter subjected to its operation; but in some cases this repulsive power of caloric will not be sufficient; for unless other substances be present to exert their attraction for the elementary or component parts of the dead mass at the same time, decomposition will not begin. On this principle we can readily understand why putrefaction may sometimes be retarded, even where air and water are in a stagnant state. In this last instance too, we are furnished with an explanation why, in some instances, both air and water may remain at rest for a length of time without becoming contaminated or proving injurious to animal life. In tropical climates, where vegetation is more luxuriant, and of course its decomposition attended with greater hazard of the accumulation of putrid particles in air and water, Nature employs stronger means of dispersion. In these regions the dews are like showers of rain; the rain like torrents; the rivers like seas; and the storms, tornadoes or hurricanes.

Thus far we have regarded water chiefly as a vehicle or transporter of dead organized matter. Its influence in promoting putrefaction falls now to be considered.

Animals and plants, when deprived of the living principle, may be preserved from decomposition in an high or low temperature of air. Flesh and fish are preserved by northern nations during Winter, by packing them in snow, without the aid of other means. This seems to be effected in consequence of the freezing of the humidity they contain, thereby preventing its decomposition and the consequent re-action of its principles on the component parts of those matters.

On the other hand, the rapid extraction of humidity from inert animal and vegetable substances by means of heat will have the same effect, of which many familiar instances might be given; and in this way the bodies of men and animals that have perished in crossing the deserts of Africa have been discovered in their natural appearance after a lapse of many years. From these observations, it would appear that the moisture contained in the remains of organized matters is the chief cause of their decomposition; this is further illustrated by the fact, that the decay of such matters immediately commences, if after having been frozen they are again thawed and exposed to a temperature but a few degrees above 32°, or when the necessary portion of water is added to such as have been dried by means of an high degree of heat. Matters preserved by drying may be transported to any other climate without undergoing any decomposition, providing they be carefully preserved from the action of the air, or insects. This may easily be effected by means of varnish.* Bodies preserved in a low tempe-

* In 1812, a young surgeon carried to sea the lower extremity of a man which had been prepared in this way in London, the leg being inclosed in a box which was put under his bed-place in his cabin. No smell was perceptible so long as the ship remained in England. On her proceeding to Lisbon, however, the doctor's secret treasure could no longer be concealed, and a ludicrous exposé took place ; but permission having been obtained to have it up in the main top, the doctor had still hopes of saving it. When it became dark, not a sailor could be found who had courage to ascend the rigging, though grog in liberal quantities was offered. The leg had, therefore, to be thrown overboard.

rature can only be kept in an atmosphere below the freezing point. The quantity of moisture present is likewise a matter of great consequence in the process of putrefaction ; for, in many instances, too much retards it. Animal bodies decay slower in a wet than in a dry grave ; and, when a dead body is immersed in water, it is converted into a substance something between wax and fat, hence called adipocire.

Although water, therefore, in a certain portion is necessary to promote putrefaction both in animal and vegetable matters, its superabundance is found to be equally powerful in preventing and restraining this process, as when it is contained in a diminished quantity. Sir John Pringle and Dr. Macbride ascertained, by experiment, that small quantities of sea salt promote the putrefactive process ; this circumstance, perhaps, admits of explanation, from the great affinity for water that subsists in the impurities with which culinary salt is always mixed, the necessary quantity of this fluid being imbibed from the atmosphere. All matters that have a strong affinity for water, as acids, alkalies, sugar, and ardent spirits, hinder putrefaction, probably by being dissolved in the humidity contained in the dead organized matter, and preventing its decomposition, although they may form new combinations with some of the other inherent principles of dead matter at the same time.

It has not been determined what precise changes the atmosphere undergoes in putrefaction ; but the powerful influence it exerts in the process cannot be doubted.

The temperature must be considerably above the freezing point (32 degrees,) but vegetables seem to require a higher temperature than animal remains ; and in either case, as before said, it is necessary it should not be so great as to cause the rapid evaporation of their humidity.

Such is a concise view of the general principles by which putrefaction is regulated. What has been said is at least sufficient to demonstrate that this important process is not left to chance, but is restrained within due bounds by the very agents which Nature employs in other circumstances to promote it. Heat promotes putrefaction, but heat also arrests its progress. Moisture promotes it, but moisture will also retard its progress. Air is necessary, but air in a state of motion is the most powerful instrument used in the prevention of the bad effects which would otherwise result from it.

The injury that would arise from the superabundance of putrid particles in the atmosphere, is prevented by other means.

Some plants come to maturity at one season, some at another, although the greatest number begins to decline in Autumn. The Winter succeeds, and hinders putrefaction from going beyond its proper limits. When it is Autumn, or the season of the greatest decay in one country, it is Winter in another. In this way dead matters undergo decomposition only in some parts of the globe at the same time, and even in the same places at different times.

The mode in which dead matters decay is not less variable.

The leaves of trees decay in a different manner from the bark, stem, or roots; the rotting of all these matters is different from that of wheat-straw. "Were the leaves when they fall," Dwight* properly remarks, " to go through the same process of fermentation and putrefaction as other vegetables, the atmosphere would be rendered so unwholesome, that it would be impossible for man either to inhabit or to clear a forested country. But the juices are exhaled before the leaves fall; they lie lightly on the ground, so as to permit a free circulation of air. So far from being offensive in their decay, they have even a peculiar fragrance, which poets have sometimes noticed among the melancholy charms of Autumn."

" The mould into which they are converted appears to be best of all manures, being united to more kinds, and producing higher degrees of vegetation than any other.

* Dwight's Travels in New England.

" This last observation accords with the experiments of Berthollet, who has shewn that, whenever the soil becomes charged with such matter, the oxygen of the atmosphere combines with it and converts it into carbonic acid gas.

" The consequence is, that the same carbon is absorbed by other vegetables, which it clothes with new foliage; these in their turn decay, and thus dissolution and renovation go on to the end of time."

During the decomposition of many vegetable substances, new products are formed, which possess properties inimical to putrefaction; salt, sugar, vinous and spirituous liquids, and acids, furnish examples of this kind; they are all powerful antiseptics, and are employed to preserve other substances from decomposition. What is still more surprising is, that the very same matters produce sugar at one stage of fermentation, wine at another, and vinegar or acetous acid at a third, according as the process is regulated with regard to heat, rest, and time.

Peat-moss is another instance of the same kind. This substance, which is only found in cold or temperate regions, is allowed on all hands to be derived from vegetable matter.

The reason why it is never found in warmer latitudes is, that the higher temperature of tropical countries promotes speedy decay, and thus prevents the necessary accumulation. It has been observed that one of the great defects of this substance as a soil is, that it is either too wet or too dry. The same property in some measure may account for its not being subject to putrefaction; but, besides this, it is known to possess peculiar antiseptic qualities which not only preserve trees and some other vegetable, but animal substances from decomposition.

Mr. Aiton, in his Treatise on Moss Earth, gives many instances of large trees having been dug out of mosses many feet deep. Some of these were afterwards used by the farmers in Scotland for roofing and flooring their houses—no small proof of their preservation, although they must have been buried for many centuries under this singular substance, as coins of the Roman Emperors, a Roman camp kettle, the sandle of a Roman soldier, an axe, &c. were found at similar depths from the surface. The axe was found near the trees which had evidently been cut down by such an instrument, as marks of the axe were observable both on the trunk and on the roots in the ground. In other instances the marks of fire were observable on both trunks and roots.

The same author likewise mentions that the body of a woman was dug out of a moss in the parish of Avondale, Lanarkshire. From the great depth at which this body was found, the slow growth, or accumulation of moss, and particularly from the circumstance of the body being covered with an antique garment of hair, it is certain that it must have been buried many centuries under this soil, yet it was in a state of good preservation. The skin was wrinkled like that of a woman after washing clothes, and the flesh pitted on pressure. When exposed to the air, however, it went into rapid decay.

Thus we see that, in whatever way we consider animal and vegetable dissolution, we must be convinced of the futility of those arguments which would persuade us that this process is generally if not always attended with danger to human health. Those who maintain such a doctrine merely from a knowledge of the fact, that all things which have ever lived must in their turns come to dissolution, might as well assert that the whole natural world is in perpetual hazard of being destroyed by caloric. Caloric is capable of consuming (as the term is) every substance in Nature ; but although it exists either in a free or latent state in all matter living or dead, yet the world is preserved from destruction by certain fixed laws : namely, that no species of matter is capable of possessing more than its share of this powerful agent ; and secondly, that the matter of heat, or the agent itself has a constant tendency to maintain an equilibrium. In a similar way all living organized matter is preserved from destruction by the decomposition of that which is dead.

Under what circumstances then let us enquire, is animal and vegetable decomposition most likely to overstep its ordinary limits.

In situations where air and water are at rest, where heat is great, and where animal and vegetable matter abounds. This brings us to the consideration of the important subject of medical topography.

The air is most likely to be stagnant in low valleys which are surrounded on every side by high mountains. In glens or gulleys, when the wind blows in certain directions. On the banks of rivers overgrown with trees, in large forests, situated on an extensive flat or plain, in the narrow crowded streets of large towns, or in hollow squares or courts surrounded with buildings. In short wherever its circulation is obstructed by any means.

The same objects which hinder the free circulation of air will often obstruct water in its course. It therefore becomes stagnant in low confined places, as in lakes, marshes, meadows, swamps, bogs, pools, ponds, ditches, ravines, gulleys, and rivers which take a long course through flat countries, and particularly in those streams which diminish greatly at one season, but overflow their banks or inundate the neighbouring country at another.

The temperature is highest within the Tropics, and vegetation is luxuriant in proportion to the richness of the soil, the degree of heat, and a due supply of moisture. Low situations are therefore rendered injurious to human health in different ways: from a richer soil, and of course greater luxuriance in vegetation; from a proper supply of moisture; and from a higher temperature and the want of a free circulation of air and water. Situation is relative or positive, neither the soil nor temperature depend so much on the positive elevation of a place above the level of the sea, as on its relative position compared with places in the immediate neighbourhood. Hence both the soil and temperature of a place are frequently materially affected by its relative position. The intervention of a mountain or forest may screen a locality from the chilling blasts of the east or north wind, or swamps and marshes, if they be situated in that direction from which the wind happens to blow a great part of the year, may render places in the neighbourhood moist and unhealthy, which would otherwise be dry and salubrious.

Water, after washing down the rich soil from the higher grounds, frequently becomes stagnant in the lower, or it deposits the alluvial soil layer upon layer. A luxuriant vegetation is the consequence, and thus all the causes of unhealthy locality become concentrated. This will depend, however, on relative position, for where the higher grounds consist of sand or gravel, the lower, instead of becoming more fertile, may be injured in this respect by the alluvial change. This seems to be one of the reasons why the soil in the immediate neighbourhood of the sea is so often found to be less productive than land which is placed at a greater distance.

If this view be correct, the opinion that animal and vegetable decomposition is most abundant on sea-coasts cannot be well founded, or at least cannot be applicable in most instances.

Again, if saline particles promote vegetable putrefaction, as some also believe, a rank growth must be the consequence; not those stunted crops generally found on the sea-coast. A light sandy and pervious soil, such as is so frequently found near the sea, can never become ostensibly marshy, although there may be transpiration of under-ground moisture; and, as the air on the sea-shore runs less danger of being obstructed than in more inland situations, we cannot tell upon what principles it should be reckoned unhealthy, except that it is on the lowest level.

On these accounts we are disposed to question the opinion, that grounds near the sea are generally more productive of marsh poison than inland districts. In other situations the explanation is easier on the principles laid down.

In rivers and running streams the rich soil taken from the

higher or neighbouring grounds by every flood is floated towards the sides or banks, where it is deposited in the form
of mud.

Sometimes it is floated by floods over the neighbouring
low grounds, where it is left on the subsiding of the water.
New pools are thus formed on the banks of rivers, and a rich
source of animal and vegetable decomposition is afforded.

Where the banks of a river are high and precipitate, confining the water within a narrow channel, of course no such
effect can be produced. Where the chief current of the
stream is in its centre, the rich soil or mud will be deposited
on both banks. If the principal current be removed by any
means from the centre to one side, or if the one is precipitate
and the other flat, one bank only will receive the deposit. If
the current be removed from the centre to both sides at the
same place, the deposit is left on the middle of the stream,
which, in course of time, may either divide it into two, or
form little islands in different parts of its course.

At the mouth of a great river a different force comes into
play.

All the soil which the river carries away is not deposited on
the banks in its course towards the ocean, but part is conveyed till the water meets with opposition from the winds,
waves, and tides. By the latter forces, a body of sand is
driven into the river's mouth. What is called a bar is thus
formed, on which the soil carried down by the river is deposited. This accumulation by degrees becomes an island,
and the river seeking new channels to disembogue itself,
several embouchures or mouths are formed.

The two celebrated rivers, the Nile and Ganges, are examples of this. The former was called Delta, from the form
of its different mouths.

The accumulation of mud and the consequent decomposition of animal and vegetable substances must therefore be
great in such situations, but we much doubt if any share of
their unhealthiness can fairly be attributed to any specific

effect produced by the mixture of the salt and fresh water. Such unhealthiness can be accounted for on ordinary principles.

In lakes, ponds, &c. the process and progress of earthy deposit are somewhat similar to what they are in running streams; the animal, vegetable, and earthy matters being washed by the waves or driven by the winds towards their margins. In proportion as this deposition accumulates vegetation increases. Aquatic herbs spring from the bottom where the lake is shallow; this affords shelter for the deposition of new matter, while decay of the herbage succeeding to growth, and growth succeeding to decay, what was at first lake, in the course of time becomes marsh or swamp, and what is swamp, gradually becomes drier till the aquatic tribe of vegetables languish for want of moisture, and leave the field to common herbage. In some places the aquatic herbage spreads along the surface of the lake in such a condensed web as to hide the water altogether. When this sward, as it is called, becomes sufficiently strong and tough to bear the human body, it obtains the name of bog. If a stick be thrust through this sward when one or two persons are upon it, the water will rise through the artificial orifice to a considerable height.

In cold and temperate regions, where the putrefactive process is slower, the accumulation of aquatic and other vegetable matter must be greater. This difference, as before said, may be one reason why peat-moss is never found in tropical climates.

It must be evident to every one that relative position is not the only thing which must be considered, in order to estimate rightly the effects likely to be produced by water in a place. Much will depend upon the soil in all the processes we have described.

If the soil be sandy, open, or pervious, the water cannot remain a sufficient length of time near the surface of the ground to form an ostensible marsh. Where the soil is clay or retentive, the water of course will readily accumulate : where the superstratum is sand or gravel, while the stratum immediately below is rock or clay, the surface of the ground will appear dry, but the under-stratum will be wet; and the moisture, being evaporated by the heat of the sun, will rise through the pervious upper-stratum. The depth of the water beneath the surface will enable us to form a pretty just estimate of the probable effects of transpiration : accordingly, Sir John Pringle, in his book on the Diseases of the Army, observes, that a deep well is one sign of a healthy locality. As putrefaction is favoured by moisture, that soil which retains the required degree longest will be most productive of animal and vegetable decomposition. If the soil be all clay it will be too retentive, and of course will be apt to become too wet. If, on the other hand, it is pervious, it will become too dry. While water falling into the cavity of a hard rock will soon be evaporated.

In a soil which is too wet the process of putrefaction is hindered; first, by the superabundant water preventing the action of the sun on the dead matter ; it is therefore subject to frequent changes of temperature. 2nd, the same cause excludes the necessary agency of the atmosphere. The effect of soil is therefore most important.

If a soil becomes too dry, putrefaction will likewise be retarded; because the attraction subsisting between the elementary principles of dead organized matter is too strong when not assisted by the joint agency of heat and moisture.— Hence, in many chemical processes, it is first necessary, in order to decompose a compound body, to lessen this attraction of its particles by pulverization, solution, and the application of heat.

The proper degree of moisture will most frequently be found on the banks of rivers, and on the margins of lakes, &c. &c.   Hence the mud found in such situations as we have described promotes putrefaction, when none happens in places where the water is sufficiently deep to exclude the action of the sun and air. From this we can readily understand why a dry season is favourable to the process in some situations, and a wet one in others; why, in the same place and in the same season, even at the same time, different degrees of putrefaction are going on, consequently why these different degrees produce different effects on the human system.

Having now explained, to the best of our understanding, the different principles connected with the operation of natutural causes upon one another, so far as they are at present known and established, we shall now proceed to make our deductions, to apply them to human health, and to enquire how far they may be fairly blamed for producing those diseases which have been usually attributed to their individual or joint operation.

The following deductions may be made from what has already been said :—

1st. As natural causes, such as air, water, caloric, &c. have no necessary connexion with the operations of man, they must have existed before man was created.

2nd. In all ages and countries they must uniformly be regulated by the same laws.

3d. Some of the natural causes must be fixed to certain localities, and cannot be removed from place to place any more than the mountains, lakes, forests, or soil, which favour their production.

4th. As marsh effluvia arise from evident objects, their presence can generally be accounted for; and the changes to which they are sometimes subject may be estimated on the same principles.

5th. They must depend on weather and season, although weather and season must have different effects according to the nature of the locality.

When the heat increases, in Spring, they will first begin to manifest themselves on the human system. As the season advances they will accumulate, as in Summer; but, in Autumn, when the temperature is not only high, but when there is a

c

greater field for animal and vegetable decomposition, they will abound most.

The succeeding Winter must check their growth. For the same reasons they must abound more in a temperate than in a cold climate, but in tropical regions most; while in those countries where there is little variation of temperature throughout the year, they will seldom if ever be totally absent.

6th. Marsh effluvia must exist in different degrees of concentration, even in the same place at the same time. No locality, therefore, of any extent, can ever generate them of the same force, or favour their accumulation to the same degree; but both must vary according to the quantity or quality of the dead organized matter, the presence or absence of moisture, the degree of heat, exposure to the air, the circulation of it, and water, &c. &c.

As all these circumstances can never be alike over a piece of ground of any extent; it is obvious that natural causes must affect the human system very differently in the same place at the same time, independent of the differences of the age, sex, or temperament of those individuals exposed to their influence; whence arise the different types or forms of a marsh disease.

7th. Marsh effluvia must be most concentrated nearest their source; they will therefore abound on low marshy confined situations, when the high, dry and better aired districts are free.

8th. For the same reasons they must be most concentrated near the surface of the earth in the mornings, before they are dissipated by the sun's heat; or in the evenings, when this heat declines, as before explained.

9th. As cultivation of the soil is nothing else than the equalization of moisture, the removal of stagnant surface water, and obstructions to the free circulation of air, the mixture of different soils together, and the appropriation of all dead organized matter to the growth of vegetables only; marsh effluvia will prevail in a country according to the state of agriculture diminishing as it advances.

10th. In countries where there is no rain for many months together, consequently where there is great want of water for agricultural and other purposes, the cultivator of the soil is forced to resort to artificial means to collect and retain it on the surface.

Under such circumstances, the diseases arising from natural causes will increase as civilization advances.

Such would be the laws of marsh effluvia if they were in any way connected with those which regulate putrefaction. Let us see how far the facts agree with the principles laid down and the deductions made from these principles.

The first settlement of all new colonies has generally been attended with the greatest sickness and mortality from climate and locality. Before ground was drained or properly cleared of wood and rank vegetation, and before dead organised matter became appropriated to the growth of living herbs and plants by the art of man, the atmosphere, in many localities, must have been much corrupted by the products of putrefaction. When countries were first settled the same motives seem to have regulated mankind in their choice of situation in all. Motives of interest more than views of health must have guided them in making this choice. Protection from wind and wave, a good supply of water and fuel, facility of land and water carriage, and a rich soil capable of cultivation, and likely to afford an abundant supply of human food, must have been the first things which would strike the first settlers on every country as being essential to their after prosperity. The mouths of great rivers or deep bays, well sheltered by high land on every side, afford the best protection from the ocean. The lee sides of mountains or of large forests give it from winds or storms of any kind, and a rich soil well supplied with water is best obtained on the banks of rivers, margins of lakes, and in low flat countries; so that we see that the very places which were first chosen as the sites of towns and new settlements were most likely to favour abundant putrefaction.

c 2

Our limits will not permit us to give a particular description of those places in different parts of the world which have been distinguished for their healthiness or unhealthiness, but the following deserve to be mentioned as illustrative of the principles we have laid down. We have visited most of them, and our opinion is, that no one who proceeds upon known principles can be much at a loss to account for the greater or less prevalence of marsh fevers in all of them.

In the East, there is Batavia, Bencoolen, Acheen, Pulo Penang, Calcutta, Trincomallee, Bombay, Point de Galle, Colomba, Madras, Diego Gascia, Bourbon, Isle of France, Cape of Good Hope, St. Helena, and Ascension.

In the West Indies, Martinique, St. Lucie, Antigua, Jamaica, St. Domingo, St. Kitt's, Nevis, Barbadoes, &c. &c.

In North America, New York, Boston, Charleston, Ballimore, New Providence, Philadelphia.

Among the islands on the way to Europe, Madeira, Teneriffe.

In Europe, Mediterranean, Levant, &c. Malaga, Carthagena, Santa Maura, Navarino, Zante, Cephalonia, Vourla, Alexandria, Smyrna, Corfu, Epidoris, Ægina, Corinth, Athens, Malta, Gibraltar, Cadiz, Lisbon.

We have particularized the above places, not so much as affording the best examples for observations on medical topography, but because they must be best known to our naval and military officers, and to the commercial world in general. Nor have we put them down in the proper order, according to their latitude or longitude. In general we have put the most unhealthy first.

According to rule, a large city situated on the marshy and woody banks of a large river, ought to be more unhealthy than one placed along an airy, open, dry, and sandy shore, where there is no river, bay, marsh, or foul beach to generate miasmata, nor woods or mountains to obstruct the ventilation or favour their accumulation. Therefore Bengal and Calcutta are more unhealthy than Madras.

A city like Batavia, which stands on the flat banks of a foul sluggish river, half choaked with mud and filth; where the principal streets are furnished with canals, the receptacles of every kind of filth and nuisance arising from a crowded population; where the mud from these canals is heaped up along the banks to dry by the heat of a vertical sun; and where at certain seasons almost every garden in the neighbourhood is converted into a marsh; ought to be more unhealthy than either Calcutta or Madras.

A harbour, formed of different deep bays, which are surrounded by jungle, marsh, and rank vegetation, and hills to obstruct the air when the wind is in certain directions, must, by the same rules, be more unhealthy than a neat clean town, situated on an open shore. Trincomallee, in the Island of Ceylon, is more unhealthy than Point de Galle or Colomba in the same island. Bombay was formerly very unhealthy, but since the evident causes of disease have been removed by draining, culture, &c. a very marked change in its salubrity has taken place.

It has been well remarked by Lind that, " in the East Indies and on the southern parts of Asia, in general, the countries which are well improved by human industry and culture, such as China, and several other places in that part of the world, are blessed with a temperate and pure air, favourable to the European constitution. On the other hand, the woody and uncultivated parts, such as the Islands of Java, Borneo, and Sumatra, the coasts of Arakan and Pegu, the islands of Negrais, where the English lately attempted to make a settlement, Banda, one of the Dutch spice islands, and several others, have proved fatal to a multitude of Europeans and others, who have been accustomed to breathe a purer air.

" In all parts of the East Indies situated near large swamps, on the muddy banks of rivers, or the foul shores of the sea, the vapours exhaling from the putrid stagnant water, whether fresh or salt, from the corrupted vegetable and the other

impurities, produce several diseases, especially during the
rainy season."

The climate of Bencoolen proved the most sickly of the
English settlements in the East. In the year 1763 many
Chinese families left Manilla in order to settle under the
English Government at this place, but most of them died
soon after their arrival. Very few of the English survived
any length of time, until they built a fort (called Fort Marl-
borough) on a dry elevated situation, at the distance of about
three miles from the town. During the rage of sickness at
Bencoolen the garrison is frequently healthy.

Bengal, next to Bencoolen, of all the English factories,
proves the most fatal to Europeans. The rainy season commences at Bengal in June and continues till October ; the
remainder of the year is healthy and pleasant. During the
rains this rich and fertile country is almost quite covered by
the overflowing of the River Ganges. Fevers, chiefly of the
remitting and intermitting kind, rage among the Europeans
in the months of July, August and September, attacking
more particularly such as are lately arrived. Sometimes
these fevers begin under a continued form, and remain several days without any perceptible remission, but they have in
general a great tendency to remission. Nor are they confined to Europeans residing there; for, in the year 1762, according to Lind, 30,000 blacks and 300 Europeans died in
the Province of Bengal. At Bombay the air is more wholesome than at Bengal, and, in general, the whole coast of
Malabar is tolerably healthy.

The Island of Bombay was improved and rendered more
healthy than it had formerly been, by building a wall to prevent the encroachment of the sea, where it formed a salt-
marsh, and by an order that none of the natives should
manure their cocoa-nut trees with putrid fish.

The rains begin here sometimes in May, but more frequently in June, and for four months are very violent.

At Surat and Tellicherry, on the same coast, Europeans commonly enjoy a good state of health.

Madras is the most healthy government belonging to the English, and in general the air of the whole coast of Coromandel is pure and salubrious when compared with most other parts of India. St. David's, Cudalore, Masulipatam, Visagapatnam, and Negapatnam, are proofs of this.

The rains do not begin on this coast until October, and continue during the months of November and December.

It is not necessary to accumulate facts to prove things which are so generally known and so universally acknowledged as what we have just stated concerning the salubrity of places in the East Indies. A few therefore will only be noticed.

" It is remarkable," says Lind, " that in the war which terminated in 1763, the English ships of war which touched at *Batavia* suffered more by the diseases of that climate (it should be locality) than they did in any other part of India, if we except a malignant scurvy which once raged in the fleet at sea. Soon after the capture of *Manilla*, the *Falmouth*, a ship of 50 guns, went to Batavia, where she remained from the latter end of July to the latter end of January, during which time she buried seventy-five of her crew, and one hundred soldiers of the 70th regiment, who were embarked on board her, not one person in the ship having escaped a fit of sickness, except her commander Captain *Brererton*.

" *The Panther*, a ship of 60 guns, was there in the years 1762 and 1764, both times unhappily during the rainy season. In the year 1762 she buried seventy of her men, and had ninety-two very ill when she left the place. In the year 1764, during a short stay, she buried twenty-five of her men. *The Medway*, which was then in company with her, lost also a great number of her men.

" The fever was of the *remitting* kind. Some were seized suddenly with a delirium, and died in the first fit. None survived the attack of a third fit."

" Nor was the fever," says the same excellent writer, " confined to the ships. The whole city afforded a scene of disease and death ; streets covered with funerals, bells tolling from morning to night, and horses jaded with dragging in hearses the dead to their graves."

We had the honour of serving in the memorable expedition to *Java*, in 1811, first on board the *Minden*, of 74 guns, and afterwards as surgeon of the *Dasher*.

The *Minden*, and several other ships of war were despatched to cruise off the island several months before the arrival of the rest of the expedition. For a considerable part of this time the Minden lay at anchor on the coast of *Bantam*, within less than half a mile's distance from the shore, and, as the Rajah of Bantam was soon gained over to the British interest, a close and frequent communication was kept up between the English and natives.

Soldiers and sailors were sent on shore to assist the natives in clearing ground for a small settlement of the latter near where the ship lay. Part of two regiments were encamped on shore along with the marines belonging to the ship, and one half of the ship's crew were sent on shore every evening, to bathe.*

---

* A few particulars concerning our camp, &c. may relieve the tiresomeness of our subject. During our stay at Bantam, a great number of the celebrated breed of cocks were sold to our sailors. As no tar, who could cut a button off an old coat was without one, a cock-pit on shore was soon formed, in which it was no uncommon thing to see twenty or thirty pair of cocks fighting in one ring. This too frequently, however, ended in a fight among the sailors themselves, every one being anxious to see fair play done his favourite sparer. These cocks were remarkably tame, and so incessant in their crowing, that they crowed as they sat on the gunwale of the boats going off to the ship, and also during the night. The noise on board being at length considered a nuisance, no more cocks were allowed to be brought or kept on board. The natives are fond of metals. On one occasion we observed one, who seemed to be a man of some consequence, with a piece of metal hanging from his neck on a string. As he seemed to value it much and to preserve it with as much care as a General

By degrees this little colony assumed more and more the appearance of an established settlement, and the presence of the Rajah and his numerous attendants and people tended to its increase. Besides our camp, temporary houses were built for the natives, and a morning and evening salute was regularly fired on shore.

Things remained in this state till our camp was suddenly attacked at day-light in the morning by a body of 600 soldiers, who had marched from Batavia for the purpose, under the command of a French Colonel. These were soon beaten off by our small party ; but as we had no particular object in view by maintaining our ground, it was judged prudent to remove it, together with the Rajah and his people, to a small island situated near the ship, and at a short distance from the main land.*

would a Waterloo gold medal, we were anxious to look at it. It turned out to be a Coventry half-penny with a hole bored through it.

One morning a signal was made on shore for a surgeon. On landing to answer it we found no less a man than the second person in rank under the Rajah himself. This high personage was called by our sailors Rajah Bagoose, which we were made to believe means Royal Highness. He conducted us to the spot where one of his men had gotten a splinter of wood run into his foot as he was assisting to clear away the bushes. We immediately extracted it and bound up the wound. This operation his Royal Highness observed with great attention, as well as examined minutely every instrument in a pocket case. His next object was to obtain some of them ; with this request we could not comply, but presented him with an old lancet, for which we were ever afterwards treated with marks of his peculiar favour.

* This was the first battle which was fought during the expedition.

Nothing could exceed the consternation of the Rajah when it began. The Dutch Government had heard of his assisting and supplying our ships, and a large sum was therefore offered for his head.

The Javanese in general are unacquainted with fire arms, though, like the Malays, they do not seem to be wanting in courage with weapons of their own choosing. The Rajah was received on board the Minden with more than usual honours. A body of marines was drawn up on the quarter-

During the time here referred to, and while the Minden's crew were employed in wooding and watering the ship, washing clothes, &c. here and in other parts of Java, they remained tolerably healthy, and but few cases of marsh remittent fever occurred on board. In many parts of the coast the water is extremely shallow at a considerable distance from the shore. The bottom in such places consists of either coral or mud. The operations of the ship were therefore difficult, as boats could not approach near the shore. On some occasions buffalo for the ship had to be drawn with ropes through this mud, with which they were completely coated before they could be got on board.

We were afterwards employed to the eastward in the *Straits of Madura,* in the Dasher. Our men, like those of the Minden, were employed on different parts of the coast, in all the operations connected with ships of war during an expedition. They were present at the taking of Samanap; yet, out of a complement of 120 men, we had seldom more than ten men on the sick-list at any time, and these chiefly with scorbutic ulcer. When we went to *Batavia,* however, the scene was soon changed, and fever and dysentery began to appear amongst the men, but chiefly those who had been on shore at this unhealthy spot.

We sailed for England with the despatches in a few days, crowded with invalids from other ships. As most of them were in a deplorable condition before we received them on board, eighteen died on the passage home, which occupied four months. A frigate which came to England soon after us, lost, we heard, thirty-two men on the passage.

We first arrived at Batavia about a month after the fall of Fort Cornelius. This we also visited.

On entering the sluggish Jucatra our attention was at once attracted by the foul and disgusting appearance of its banks.

deck, who were directed to fire a volley over his head when he appeared on board. This he did not seem to like.

In many parts the corrupting offals of animal and vegetable putrefaction were so evident, that few persons would have liked to wash their hands in the almost stagnant water : for, even at this time, several human bodies were seen floating amongst the rank vegetation which fringes its banks, although so long a period had elapsed since any fighting had taken place.

The city of Batavia has a gay and even elegant appearance ; like some other Dutch towns, canals run in the direction of the principal streets. Over these, elegant bridges are thrown, and rows of evergreens are planted at equal distances along their banks.

We were conducted to a large hotel, where the English, French, and Dutch officers were living together in the greatest harmony.*   A Malay band of music belonging to one of the regiments attended for their amusement; loyal toasts were given by the officers of the three nations indiscriminately ; and whether the band struck up " God save the King," or " Buonaparte's march," it was received with the same respect by every one present.

The barracks, in which the principal body of troops are quartered, are placed at *Weltervreeden*, about three miles distant. This place we were told is healthy, but a single glance at the inhabitants is sufficient to do away with the first impressions of a stranger on entering Batavia. The squalid and anxious look, the sallow complexion and meagre form of almost every one you see cannot be mistaken. You can

* During our stay at Batavia, we were accosted by a lady who was walking with a Dutch officer; she was anxious to inform us that she was born in London—" my father Sir is still there, probably you may have heard his name ? he lives in Treadneedle-street." An address so unusual in such a place naturally led to farther explanation. She had left England when a child, was married to the officer, a Gorman, with whom she had lived chiefly in the Dutch foreign settlements. This may account for the simplicity of the question, and her total ignorance of Europe, and London, her native city.

scarcely pass along a street, or enter a place or square without meeting a hurling chair, not containing a child surrounded with toys, but an adult supported by cushions or pillows. The same emaciated objects may be frequently seen sitting in an easy chair under the shade of the trees, or in the balconies in front of the houses. The canals mentioned above have been covered over with the best effects.

Bengal must next occupy our attention. Dr. James Johnson, speaking of the endemic or marsh remittent fever of Bengal, says, the importance of this disease will not be questioned, when it is considered that, in the small portion of the Hoogly, running between Calcutta and Kedgere, full three hundred Europeans (better than a fourth of the ship's crew) fall annual victims to its ravages. This immense river (Ganges) originating in the mountains of Tibet, and winding in a south-eastern direction, collecting its tributary streams from all quarters as it proceeds, after a course of more than a thousand miles, bursts its boundaries in the rainy season, and covers the plains of Bengal with an expansive sheet of turbid water. But the ground springing a little as it approaches the coast, prevents the inundation from rushing at once into the ocean; it therefore disembogues itself slowly through a multiplicity of channels that intersect the great Indian Delta, or Sunderbunds, in every possible direction.

This check keeps the plains of Bengal overflowed from the latter end of July till the middle of October; during which period, noted cities, populous villages, exalted mosques, and stupendous pagodas, are seen just above the level of the temporary ocean, surrounded by innumerable boats, now the habitations of domesticated animals.

At this time vessels even of a hundred tons are beheld traversing the country in various routes, wafted by a breeze that seldom shifts more than a point or two from South. The depth of water, during the inundation, varies from ten to thirty feet, according to the undulations of the ground.

The original course of rivers is now known only by their currents, which may have a velocity of four miles an hour on an average : while the great body of water spread over the plains, moves at the rate of half a mile or a mile in the same space of time.

It would be endless to trace all the sources of pollution in the vegetable and mineral kingdoms. One or two only in the animal kingdom will be selected as specimens in that extensive department.

The Hindoo religion enacts that, as soon as the spirit has taken its departure, the body shall be burnt on the banks of the Ganges, and that the ashes, together with every fragment of the funeral pile, be committed to the sacred stream. In a country where dissolution and putrefaction are nearly simultaneous, the utility of such a measure is self-evident, but, either from indolence or penury, the body is now generally placed on a small hurdle, and when little more than scorched is pushed off from the shore, with a bamboo, there to float, until it arrives at the ocean, unless it be previously picked up by a shark or alligator ; or, which is frequently the case, dragged on shore by Pariar dogs, and devoured by them, in company with a numerous train of carrion birds of various descriptions. From one hundred to one hundred and fifty of these disgusting objects may be counted passing any one point in the course of a day ; and in some places where eddies prevail, a whole vortex of putrid corses may be seen circling about for hours together. It was very common for us to be obliged to " clear cable" occasionally of a human body, speckled over by the partial separation of the cuticle from putrefaction.

Each contributary stream brings down its full proportion of these ingredients to the general reservoir ; since the inland inhabitants have always recourse to that which is most contiguous to their village, and strange as it may appear, where no stream is at hand, the nearest tank or jeel performs the

office of the sacred Ganges; supplying drink for the living
and a final receptacle for the dead. We may add, that the
banks of this river present, particularly about the rising and
setting of the sun, a motley group of all classes, and sometimes both sexes, sacrificing to the goddess Cloacina in collo-
quial association; not indeed offering their gifts in temples,
but committing them freely to the passing current.

The same author also observes, that the more complete
the inundation, the more healthy are the inhabitants, till the
fall of the waters in November and December, exposes a
number of miry and slimy marshes to the action of a still
powerful sun, when those who are in their neighbourhood, are
sure to come in for a share of remittents and intermittents.

The Sunderbunds, and the country for some way round
Calcutta, being in most places rather above the level of high-
water mark, become, during the rainy season, an immense
woody and jungly marsh, neither perfectly overflowed, nor
yet quite dry—in a word, presenting a surface as well supplied with animal and vegetable matters in a state of decomposition, and combining all the other circumstances necessary
for giving miasmata their full influence on the human body,
viz. intense heat, moisture, calms, &c. as perhaps any spot of
equal extent on the face of the globe.

These Sunderbunds form a belt between the Hoogly and
the Magna of about 180 miles in length by 50 in depth,
completely overrun with forests, underwood, and jungle, and
inhabited by animals of various species, who are left to the
uninterrupted possession of this frightful territory.

The inhabitants and domesticated animals of inundated
districts, are all this time cooped up in a state of torpor; but
at Calcutta and Diamond Harbour it is far otherwise. There,
the Europeans are not confined, and business must be attended to as much as during the dry or the cool and healthy
season. It will not, therefore, appear extraordinary that, under all circumstances related, the marsh remittent fever should

make such ravages among all classes, but more particularly among those who are exposed to the sultry heat of the day, the rains, the dews, and intemperance.*

The above account of Bengal we have taken from one of our best authors on tropical climates. He has given a very lively, and, we believe, a faithful account of the causes of remittent fever, and the general unhealthiness of this presidency. Surely nothing more than what we have extracted from his work was required to account for both. It therefore gives us pain to be obliged to add, that the same respectable writer has travelled so far out of his way as the moon in order to elucidate his subject. What he has said upon this luminary appears to be but reflected light.

It is not necessary to enlarge on the medical topography of India and the East, for the purpose of proving what has been said ; namely, that motives of interest, more than any other, have generally directed European nations in the choice of foreign settlements. The two great capitals we have described are melancholy instances of the fact. Little have the two Governments of England and Holland reflected on the subject. We hear of the prizes it is true, but the blanks are for ever buried in oblivion.

The settlements of the different European nations on the West coast of Africa exhibit convincing proofs of the same kind. The part of the coast here referred to extends from Cape de Verd, in 15° North lat. and 16° West long. to Cape Formoso, in lat. 4° North and 5° West long., comprehending a line of coast of upwards of two thousand miles.

The Portuguese navigators were the first who explored this part of Africa, about the middle of the 15th century ; but the French, English, Dutch, and Danes, have all had possessions on this coast since that time.

The principal forts and settlements are *St. Mary's, Sierra Leone, Apollonia, Axim, Hollandia, Dixcove, Succumbee,*

---

* See Johnson on Tropical Climates.

Commenda, St. George del Mino, Anamaboo, Cape Coast Castle, St. Paul de Loanda, St. Salvadore, and Goree.

We shall not attempt to give a particular description of these different places, nor is this requisite, as they present a sameness of character peculiar to all flat, woody and uncultivated countries, and all of them, except the last, are situated either on the banks of rivers or on the shores of the Atlantic. A general description of the country will therefore suffice. Its situation; the number of its rivers, lakes, and marshes; its soil, climate, uncultivated condition, and general aspect; with the savage state of its native population, all conspire to render it unhealthy, and leave nothing to conjecture as to the causes of those diseases for which it has long been remarkable.

" The first novelty," says a late writer[*], " that strikes the visitor of the African coast, is its extreme lowness. The earliest indication of its approach will be afforded him by the temperature of the sea diminishing considerably, even before the seaman's plummet has declared the depth of the water. Its depth begins gradually to lessen, and at length the soundings are reduced to ten or twelve fathoms. The land at last appears, the tops of trees appear to emerge out of the water towards the eastern horizon, and in a few hours the appearance of a dense and nearly level forest indicates its near approach. While advancing towards the coast, or sailing in its parallel, the nights are enlivened by the constant flashes of lightning upon the land; or, when at too great a distance to descry it, they are seen gleaming in constant succession towards that quarter of the horizon in which it lies."

This description is not applicable to a few places on the coast only; for, excepting the mountains about Sierra Leone, and here and there a small eminence or hill, the whole of the coast presents nearly the same aspect; and in several parts

---

[*] See Quarterly Journal of Foreign Medicine and Surgery, for January, 1821.

the flatness extends even into the interior of the country, to the distance of some hundreds of miles.

The country is watered by innumerable *rivers* and *rivulets,* which traverse it in almost every part. Some of these take their rise in the King and other mountains in the interior of Africa; and, running a long course through a low flat country, disembogue themselves into the Atlantic ocean.

The *Gambia, Rio Grande, Sierra Leone, Congo, Senegal, Rio Nunes, Pongos* and *Dembia,* are the chief rivers which take this course.

As most of the great rivers, and even rivulets, overflow their flat banks, and inundate the country at certain seasons to a great extent, while they are much dried up, or narrowed in their breadth at others, the quantity of mud and ooze which they leave upon the ground, exposed to the action of a burning sun, is very great, besides converting nearly the whole country into swamps and marshes.

The *soil* is the most favourable for forming these. In most places it is deep, rich, and fertile; owing to evident causes. Where it is not sandy it is a loamy clay, or rich black mould. Even where the upper stratum is sand, there is a retentive clayey or rockey bottom. In some places a heavy clay soil extends to within a few yards of the sea.

The *climate* is likewise favourable to animal and vegetable decomposition for the most part of the year; the heat being sometimes as high as 100°, but never descending below 83°. At St. Mary's, on the Gambia, the nature of the soil and its less dense vegetation render, at some seasons, the degree of heat frequently greater than in most of the other settlements on the coast; and, when the sun has considerably passed the equator towards his greatest northern declination, the thermometer in the shade has frequently indicated upwards of 100°. The temperature of the air at Sierra Leone is somewhat lower, being not more than 95°; but its tranquil state, with regard to its horizontal motion, favours the multiplication of the foreign ingredients derived from the soil and deeaying vegetation ; consequently the atmosphere in this state feels very sultry and oppressive. The mean temperature observed at different periods of the day throughout the year, was from 83° to 83½°.

The *seasons* are divided into the rainy and dry. The former, generally speaking, lasts between four and five months. At Sierra Leone the rains begin in June, and end with October ; while at Gambia, they commence a fortnight or three weeks sooner than at Senegal. Down the coast their commencement becomes more early as the latitude decreases.

The *quantity of rain* which falls during the rainy season, almost exceeds belief. By observations made at Senegal, 115 inches depth of rain were found to fall in four months ; a quantity equal to that which falls in England during the space of four years. It has been observed, that the number of days of rain diminish as we approach the equator, while the quantity of rain that annually falls increases ; but, owing to the locality of Sierra Leone, says the writer before quoted, the moisture being attracted by the hills and mountains in its neighbourhood, the actual number of days in which rain falls there, is greater than in most northern climates.

By a register, he says, kept in this colony, the number of rainy days amounted to 204, and of the remaining dry days, although the moisture of the atmosphere was not actually condensed into rain, yet the greater number of them exhibited its progress towards that state; not only the adjoining mountains, but the river and its banks being covered with fogs and haze. The rainy season, which begins with June and ends with October, as before said, is both introduced and closed by tornados. The number of tornados, by an account kept during one whole year, amounted to fifty-four; no part being more obnoxious to them than this and the Grain Coasts.

Thunder and lightning are of frequent occurrence here, as they also are along the whole coast.

The *winds*, during the rains, generally blow from the Southwest, or West-south-west. About their commencement, and after their conclusion, the atmosphere is generally tranquil. At other seasons, the sea and land winds occur, but not in regular succession. The sea-breeze seldom appears, and when it does, it generally dies away in a few hours, leaving the air sultry and stagnant. The land winds come on about sun-set, and only amount to very light breezes; and, from blowing over the adjoining woods and swamps, are generally a source of disease.*

Lind, in speaking of Guinea, says, "the soil is either marshy or watered with rivers or rivulets, whose swampy or oozy banks are overgrown with sedges, mangroves, and the most noxious weeds, the slime and filth on which, send forth an intolerable stench, especially towards the evening. At a distance, this extensive coast appears in most places flat and covered with low suspended clouds. On a nearer approach, there are generally perceived heavy dews, which fall in the night; and the land is every morning and evening wrapped up in a fog. Upon examining the face of the country, it is found clothed with a perpetual and pleasant verdure, but altogether uncultivated, excepting a few spots which are generally surrounded with forests or thickets of trees, impenetrable to refreshing breezes, and fit only for the resort of wild beasts.

"It is not uncommon," he adds, "in many trading factories, to meet with a few Europeans, pent up in a small spot of low, damp ground, so entirely surrounded with thick woods, that they can scarcely have the benefit of walking a few hundred yards, and where there is not so much as an avenue cut through any part of the woods for the admission of wholesome and refreshing breezes. The Europeans have also unfortunately fixed some of their principal settlements on low, inland, and ulcultivated spots on the foul banks, or near the swampy and oozy mouths of rivers, or on salt marshes, formed by the overflowing of the ocean; where, in many places, the

* See Foreign Journal.

putrid fish, scattered on the shore by the negroes, emit such noisome effluvia as prove very injurious to health.

Notwithstanding what has been said, I think it will hardly admit of a doubt, that if any tract of land in Guinea was as well improved as the Island of Barbadoes, and as perfectly freed from trees, underwood, marshes, &c. the air would be rendered equally healthful there, as in that pleasant West Indian Island."—*Lind on Hot Climates.*

According to the same author, the most healthy place, or the Montpellier, for its air, of the Portuguese settlements in that division of the globe, is the town of St. Salvadore. Notwithstanding this lies 150 miles up the river Congo or Zaire, and within six degrees of the equator, yet, from its being situated on a hill, and the neighbouring country being cleared of the natural woods and thickets, its inhabitants breathe a temperate and pure air, and are, in a great measure, exempted from all the plagues of an unhealthy climate.

Cape Coast Castle, the principal settlement belonging to this country, on the contrary, stands on a very low and insignificant prominence of granite and quartz rocks. The native town is placed near the walls of the castle between it and the adjoining country. The town is built of the tenacious and heavy clay which forms the soil on which it stands, and the houses are so closely placed to each other as scarcely to admit a passage between them : during the rainy season every house appears placed in a mire of clay and mud. In every considerable vacancy, and on the grounds immediately surrounding the town, accumulations of every species of filth would soon take place, did not the moist and warm atmosphere promote its decomposition and carry off the volatilized products, while insects, reptiles, and birds, assist in furthering the same effect.

We shall finish what we have got to add regarding the medical topography of this quarter of the world, by inserting a letter from our friend John Shower, Esq. late colonial surgeon at Sierra Leone. This gentleman, after having served ten years there in the above capacity, had to return home from impaired health, but not without receiving the handsomest testimonials, and two rewards from mercantile bodies, for his humanity and attention.

Dear Sir,

I was at Sierra Leone from the year 1816 until the year 1826, with the exception of a few months on sick-leave in 1819, during which term I had frequent opportunities of seeing the fever of that climate. The troops laying there were the Royal African Corps, and depôt of the 2d West India Regiment, which were native as well as English. They were generally stationed in Fort Thornton, about a quarter of a mile from the town. The soil in the environs of Sierra Leone is chiefly clay and rock, which, although not very deep, is extremely fertile, and vegetation very luxuriant. The ground is in general high and mountainous. The mountains are covered with high trees and impenetrable underwood : in fact, the whole neighbourhood seems a large forest. The banks of the river are clean. The rainy season commences about June and continues until the month of October or beginning of November. During my stay there, my duty was that of colonial surgeon, as well as apothecary to the forces. We had fevers every day, during my stay, throughout the whole year; but, during the rainy season, the number of my patients was seldom less than thirty or forty, including natives and Europeans, per diem. The type of fever was either of the bilious remittent kind or intermittent, but mostly the former. Strangers did not seem to be more susceptible of it than those who had been there some time; but when attacked generally it proved fatal. As the natives usually employ their own remedies, I had not much opportunity of ascertaining the exact proportion of them which were attacked with these fevers; but I am perfectly certain they suffer every year to a certain degree, though in a milder form. The black population consists of Maroons from Jamaica, and Nova Scotian settlers, and liberated Africans. All of the former two have been long settled, and have families grown up since their settlement.

The fever, during the rainy season, was the severest form of what is called marsh fever, frequently proving fatal in five or seven days, but it often continued for weeks, and when that was the case the patient generally recovered. The form in the beginning of the milder cases was frequently intermittent, assuming the remittent type after a few paroxysms. Second and third attacks were so common as almost to be *universal*. On dissection, no particular morbid appearances were observed, except invariably enlarged *spleen* to a great extent, weighing some pounds—in one, I think, 7¼. The general treatment was by opening the bowels with calomel and jalap, and, during the febrile attacks, administering the effervescing draught with ammon. carbonat., and when a remission took place, giving the cinchona quinine; but I have never seen any good from the use of the lancet; on the contrary, where the lancet has been resorted to, the patients, if they recovered, it was but slowly, and almost invariably became œdematous or anasarcous. Mercury was always given in doses of three or four grains every two or three hours, until the mouth became sore, and with decided advantage.

During my ten years' stay at Sierra Leone, I never saw any other fever, but in 1823, when a fever broke out there similar to the yellow fever of the West Indies, attended with black vomit, which was supposed to have been brought there from the Mediterranean by a ship called the Caroline ; this I recognized as a different fever from the one I have just described from the common fever of the country, and, to my knowledge, none of the medical men then at Sierra Leone had any difficulty in distinguishing it as a new and different disease.

The harbour-master, who was the first who visited the Caroline, was the first who was attacked and died of black-vomit :—he had been in Sierra Leone and on the coast for about seven years. It is worthy of remark, that this fever only attacked the Europeans and not the blacks. This was about the latter end of March or beginning of April, when the common fever of the country was not prevalent, and be-ing the finest part of our season. The mortality was almost universal in those it attacked—out of my own patients there were only five or six survived. The form of this fever par-took of the continued type, and never of the remittent or in-termittent. Black vomit was observable in every case that died. Only two of our medical staff escaped an attack—all those that were attacked died. I have my doubts whether it was imported or contagious—I am much of opinion that it pro-ceeded from the atmosphere, although the weather was not different either in point of temperature, moisture, or prevail-ing winds, nor was there any difference observable in the nature of the locality, the crops, or general health of the people, from what it is usually at this season. I have since heard that a similar fever, attended with black vomit, made its appearance in 1828, after my departure, which attacked natives and Europeans indiscriminately. The fever of 1823 disappeared soon after the rainy season commenced.

I am,

Dear Sir,

Your obedient Servant,

JOHN SHOWER.

Late Colonial Surgeon, Sierra Leone.

To Dr. Aiton, Surgeon, R.N.
Malta, 27th July, 1830.

In such countries as we have just described, cultivation is all that is wanted to render them healthy. It is in those which are long without rain, and where the ground becomes parched by the heat of a powerful sun, during certain seasons, that cultivation proves injurious to human health. The cul-tivators of such soils being obliged to obviate the want of moisture by artificial means, the water of the smallest streams is spread over the neighbouring grounds, to irrigate the land; or sometimes several rivulets are collected into one, to drive a mill, or form ponds for different purposes. In Greece, such instances abound; particularly about *Athens, Epidaurus, Corinth,* and *Patras.* There, the water-courses assume the appearance of regular formed roads, in the dry season, and the traveller is undeceived by the wooden bridges that sometimes interrupt his progress, or by small pools of stagnant water.

The general arid aspect of such countries has often misled the casual observer into a belief of their healthiness.

Several instances of a similar kind may be met with in *New England,* but with this difference; that here, mill-ponds are formed.

But the *Campagna de Roma* affords a still more striking example of this.

Professor Koreff, (as well as all who have written on the same subject) gives a striking picture of the livid unhealthiness of its miserable inhabitants. Miserable, however, as may be their condition, it does not present half so heart-rending a picture, as that of the ill-fated natives of *Basse, Bresse, Brenne, Sologna,* &c.

The mode of cultivating the land in these districts consists in forming it alternately into ponds, and then submitting it to tillage; it is kept in the state of ponds for 18 months, or two years; at the expiration of which, the water is made to run into a neighbouring field : the land is recultivated for one or two years, and afterwards again formed into ponds. Added to the ponds and marshes, there are also numerous woods, which surround the humid plains, and intercept the circulation of air; the consequence of this is, that the whole country is almost uninhabited. The labourers enter into the wet land soon after it is drained, in order to put it into a state of culture, and pass whole days up to mid-leg in humidity, imbibing the pestiferous exhalations at every pore.

" Il est rare," says M. Foderè, " que de quatre travailleurs deux n'y succombent."—See *Foderè's works, and Quarterly Review*, vol. XXVIII.

In countries naturally dry, *a wet season* is unfavourable to health ; whereas, in wet soils, a dry season is the most injurious. The reason of this has been already explained.

Many proofs of the fact are mentioned by Lind, and other writers on marsh fever. On the west coast of Africa, and in Barbadoes, Antigua, and some other West Indian islands, which are liable to long droughts, like the countries we last described, marsh fevers occur very seldom in those dry seasons, but they become very prevalent whenever these droughts are suddenly terminated by much rain.

A *dry season*, on the other hand, is favourable to putrefaction in all countries, which, from their lowness, are frequently inundated with water. It is not when they are overflown that this happens, but when the soil is left in a state just sufficiently moist. The Dutch and French colonies, on the coast of Guiana, as *Surinam*, also, *Berbice, Demerara, Essequebo*, as well as *Cayene*, and the adjoining settlements on the continent, some parts of the islands of *Martinico, Dominico*, and *St. Domingo*, in the West Indies, (and many others might be mentioned) are instances of this kind.

In some situations the *first rains* of the season have been observed to have a bad effect in producing marsh fevers. This cannot proceed from the putrefaction of animal and vegetable substances existing in the soil at the time ; for this, being a slow process, even under the most favourable circumstances of heat, moisture, air, and rest, we cannot believe that water, suddenly applied in the form of rain, could cause decomposition in a short time. The fact, however, may be otherwise explained. The products of putrefaction which were previously mixed with the soil, or pent up, as it were, by the dry weather, may be again disengaged or let loose by the first rains. Still it must appear evident, that miasmata, arising from such a source, must be very limited in duration ; for, whenever the upper stratum was washed by the rains, and the atmosphere cleared of foreign matters floating in it, the effects would cease till the new products of putrefaction were formed by that degree of moisture which is favourable to decomposition. We have observed a sudden change from dry to wet weather to produce a few cases of marsh-fever on board of ship, where putrid particles could not be fairly suspected. As such cases generally occur in those persons who have had a former attack of the disease, it seems probable that the sudden change of weather acts as an exciting cause only, consequently that it operates on the living body which has been previously exposed to the action of miasmata in some other place, and not upon dead organized matters, or the products of putrefaction in any shape.

In treating of medical topography, the effects of woods and hills on miasmata must not be forgotten. Woods have sometimes a good and sometimes a bad effect on human health. According to several writers, wherever marshes are situated near a great city, the intervention of wood must necessarily form a screen to impede the wafting of miasmata by the winds. Perhaps this might have been the reason why the ancients consecrated the woods in the vicinity of Rome to Neptune, in order to secure them from the axe; in the distresses, however, in which the great expenditure of Pius VI. involved the holy see, a large district of these woods had been sold and cut; and to this event, Sir Charles Morgan thinks, may, with some reason, be attributed an increase of danger to the unprotected city. The evils resulting from cutting woods under the circumstances above alluded to, are strongly exemplified in a Memoire on the Physical Properties of Malaria, by M. Rigaud de l'Isle, and inserted in the Bibliotheque Universale for May, 1817. The following are his examples.

Near St. Stephens, on Mount Argentel, a convent is situated, which was famed for the salubrity of its air; but since the forests which surrounded it have been cleared, it has become unhealthy.

At Velletri, near the Pontine marshes, the cutting down intermediate wood occasioned immediately, and for three successive years, fevers and other diseases which committed great ravages. The same effects were observed from a similar cause near Campo Salino, and analogous examples might be adduced from Volney, Lancisi, Donas, and others.—*Vid. Quar. Rev. Vol.* 28.

Mountains will have a similar good effect in some situations.

" It may, at first sight, appear singular," says Dr. James Johnson, "that mountainous countries covered with lofty woods or thick jungle should give rise to fevers similar, in every respect, to those of flat and marshy districts. But the reason is obvious when we consider that, in the first-mentioned situations, the surface of the earth is constantly strewed, particularly in Autumn, with vegeto-animal remains, and kept in a moist state by the rains or drippings of dews from the superincumbent foliage. The stratum of atmosphere, therefore, in contact with the ground, becomes highly impregnated with effluvia, which are seldom agitated by breezes or rarified by the rays of the sun, either of which would tend to dissipate the exhalations. Thus, amongst the lofty forest and impenetrable jungles of Ceylon, the most powerful miasmata are engendered, producing fevers of great violence and danger."—*Vid. Lord Valentia's Travels, Vol.* 2d.

It has been observed that Pennsylvania is now more unhealthy than formerly; that bilious and remittent fevers, which a few years appeared chiefly in the neighbourhood of rivers, creeks, and mill-ponds, now appear in parts remote from them all, and *in the highest situations.* This change has been traced to three causes;—1st. To the increase of mill-ponds. Till these were established, intermittents in several countries in Pennsylvania were unknown. 2d. To clearing the country. A distinction, however, is to be made between clearing and cultivating a country ; while clearing a country makes it sickly in the manner that has been mentioned, cultivating a country, that is, draining swamps, destroying weeds, burning brushwood, and exhaling the superincumbent and unwholesome moisture of the earth, by means of frequent crops of grain, grasses, and vegetables of all kinds, renders it healthy. The 3d cause mentioned is, the immense quantities of rain which had fallen when the above observations were made by Dr. Rush.—*Rush's Enquiries.* Dr. Hunter, in his book on the Diseases of the Army in Jamaica, p. 15, observes—" In dry sandy spots, nearly surrounded by the sea, there is little or no decay of vegetable or animal matter, and there is no moisture, for the rain is immediately absorbed by the sand; such places, therefore, are healthy, and almost exempt from fevers. *Elevated and mountainous situations are also healthy;* for what there is of decayed vegetable and animal matter is washed away by the frequent rains, which do not penetrate the ground, but, in running off, carry whatever is light and loose along with them. What is thus carried off is frequently deposited in the valleys among the hills, but these are so small, that they do not form a bottom large enough to emit vapours hurtful in any great degree ; add to this, that the inhabitants never set down their houses in such bottoms, but constantly make choice of lofty situations. *How much it contributes to health, being raised even a little above* the exhalation, may be judged from this ; that, in the flat parts of the country, the houses upon a level with the ground, or but little raised above it, are uniformly the most unhealthy."

Having now finished our observations on medical topography in general, pointed out the localities most favourable to the generation of miasmata, and also explained the agency of different natural causes, with the share each have in their production, it is necessary to say something regarding the physical properties of these noxious effluvia.

1st. The specific gravity of marsh or marsh-like miasmata is greater than that of atmospheric air.

Dr. James Clark, in his Medical Notes on Climate, &c. mentions circumstances communicated to him by Professor Brera, whilst attending the clinical wards of the hospital at Padua. "The wall of that wing of the building where these wards are situated is washed by a branch of the sluggish Brenta, and it frequently happened that the windows of them, which were about sixteen feet from the surface of the water, having been carelessly left open until too late an hour, several of the patients were attacked with intermittent fevers, in some instances of the pernicious kind. This never occurred in the women's ward, which are immediately over those of the men, though there is no reason to believe that more care was taken in shutting the windows of those than of the latter."

The Baron de Humboldt observed that the farm of Eucero, situated above Vera Cruz, is a stranger to the insalubrity which reigns over the whole coast. The elevation of this farm being 3015 feet, no conclusion can be drawn from this fact, nor from the following:—M. Regaud de l'Isle, by observations made in the neighbourhood of Rome, tried to fix the point at which the marsh effluvia are innocuous; this he considers to vary from 682 to 1006 feet above the level of the place whence they emanate. "Ghent," says Sir J. Pringle, "is situated between the high and low division of Flanders. One part of the town, called St. Peter's Hill, is much higher than the rest, and in this, the barracks, having drains and free air, were quite dry, so that the soldiers who lay there enjoyed perfect health; but those who were quartered in the lower parts of the town, mostly in the ground-floors of waste-houses, unprovided with drains, and of course damp, were sickly. The battalion of the 1st Regiment of Guards was an instance of the effect of this difference of quarters. Two of the companies lay on St. Peter's Hill, the remaining eight in the lower parts of the town, in rooms so very damp, that the men could scarce keep their belts and shoes from moulding. In the month of July the sick of this battalion amounted to about one hundred and forty;—only two men belonged to the garrison on the hill, and the rest to those of the lower town."—*Page* 12. Similar observations have been made in other parts of the world.

Dr. Hunter, in his work on Diseases of the Army in Jamaica, page 306, says, " the barracks of Spanish Town, consists of two floors ; the first upon the ground, the second on the first. The difference in the health of the men in the two floors was so striking as to engage the attention of the assembly of the Island of Jamaica ; and, upon investigation, it appeared that three were taken ill on the ground floor, for one in the other. The ground floor was not, therefore, used for a barracks afterwards."

Mr. Ralph, assistant surgeon of 2d Queen's Regt., has given, in the Medico-Chirurgical Transactions, vol. VIII, page 70, a report which illustrates the same facts in a striking manner. "By a calculation made in this report, on the health of the men at Basse Terre Gaudalope, it appears, that in the month of August, one case of fever presented itself in every twentieth man of those quartered on the ground-floor; and in each thirteenth man of those on the upper floor. During that part of the month of September which has elapsed, each twenty-fourth man was attacked with fever of those stationed in the upper room, and each fourteenth among those in the lower."

" It is very rare," says Dr. Furgerson, "to hear of an ague occurring in the sea-port town of Basse Terre Guadalope, either amongst the troops there or inhabitants ; but in the barracks, on the cool *marshy* hills above the town, at an elevation of less than 1000 feet, it was a very common disease, both amongst the officers and soldiers, while their comrades of the same corps, in the barracks of the town, suffered from the more concentrated forms of remittent fever alone.

" The same may be said of nearly the whole of the West

India towns. They are all so marshy that, in colder latitudes, they could not possibly escape being infected with agues ; but these very seldom originate, and are nearly unknown amongst them. It is common to hear the inhabitants of Barbadoes boast that an ague cannot be found in their island, although they have various marshes, particularly near Bridgetown, and, during sickly seasons, come in for their share of yellow fever. The reason is plain ; there are very few ridges of sufficient elevation, and their sides are not marshy, but dry calcareous strata.

"It has commonly been remarked," says the same author, "that when the garrison of the lofty position of Morné Fortuné is healthy, during the fine dry weather, the inhabitants of the town of Castrus, at the base of the same hill immediately below, within half common shot, are visited by the worst fevers, and vice versâ. The dry weather gives activity to the miasmata which the rains dilute, refresh, or condense, at the same time that they are forming pools or temporary swamps on the shoulders of the hill, immediately beneath the barracks on the summit of Morné Fortuné."

The evidence as to the distance to which malaria proves injurious, in a perpendicular direction, seems rather contradictory; for, while some authors assert that a height of twenty feet greatly diminishes its power, others adduce proof of its being attracted by hills of the elevation of 1000 feet. We have the very high testimony of Sir Gilbert Blane, in favour of the latter opinion, who gives Northfleet as an instance, where the high grounds were infested, while the low marshy places, in the same neighbourhood, were free. Dr. Maton points out instances of the same kind in the neighbourhood of Weymouth. The opinion of M. Rigaud, on the same subject has already been given, and Dr. James Johnson says, " there can be no doubt that hills and mountains arrest the course of miasmata through the air, and, when a sufficient quantity of them is collected, they will produce their effects on the human frame in a similar manner, as if issuing from

48   DISSERTATIONS ON HEALTH.

their original source, *especially when the predisposing causes are in great force.* Hence we see how miasmal fevers may take place on the summit of Morné Fortuné, or the Rock of Gibraltar, without any necessity for supposing that the febrific exhalations arose from these places themselves."—*On Climate.*

Dr. Hunter, on the other hand, observes, "how much it contributes to health, being raised even *a little above* the exhalations." And a host of evidence corroborating his observation might easily be added. How, then, is this disparity to be reconciled? How is a sufficient quantity of miasmata to be collected on the summits of Morné Fortuné and the Rock of Gibraltar, to produce their effects on the human frame, as Dr. Johnson imagines?

An explanation of the former has been given by Dr. Bancroft in his essay on Yellow Fever, p. 231:—"When the small elevation of a single story (not exceeding 20 feet)" says the Dr. "from the ground, is found greatly to diminish the power of noxious exhalations, it might be expected, that the tops of hills, rising a few hundred feet above the level of the sea, or of the surrounding country, would always be found healthy. Experience, however, has often proved the contrary, particularly on the Morné Fortuné, at St. Lucie, and on the Hospital and Richmond Hill, at Grenada; where very great mortality has repeatedly occurred among British soldiers. But in these, and similar cases, it seems probable that *the soil, at or near the tops of these hills,* contained matters suited to the formation of marsh miasmata, with sufficient proportions of clay to retain the necessary moisture. *There can, indeed, be no doubt that this is the case of the Morné Fortuné,* which I observed to be *very wet, and in some degree swampy.* This and Richmond Hill, being at their tops more than 700 feet above the level of the sea, *could not, I am persuaded, be so greatly affected merely by exhalations from any low and damp grounds in their neighbourhood.*"

A similar explanation has been given of the mountains in

Ceylon, by Lord Valentia, as before quoted by Dr. Johnson. But the rock of Gibraltar has no swamp on its summit to engender miasmata, no clay to retain the necessary moisture, no trees, jungle, or brush-wood, to collect them, no lurking place to protect their slender frames from "the rainy Levanter, that makes even stones to canter."* The rock is about 1,000 feet above the level of the sea, and is nearly insulated, being miles distant from any marshy lands. The force of attraction would therefore require to be very great ; 1st, to bring the miasmata from so great a distance ; 2nd, to elevate them to so great a height ; and lastly, make them hold on the rock with the force of muscles or other shell-fish.

It is not improbable, however, that, in cases where mountains *are surrounded closely on every side by an immense tract* of flat marshy country, as in some parts of the Campagna di Roma, unhealthy exhalations may find their way to the height of 1,000 feet, in the manner Sir Gilbert Blane describes. That very respectable writer says, " Water recently exhaled from the surface of the earth has a tendency to ascend, and being lifted over parts on the same level, impinges on the neighbouring heights. The watery vapours prove a vehicle of unwholesome volatile matters, which, after ascending, are attracted by hills like clouds." Still we are without proof, and can only judge by effects ; but as these effects are somewhat ambiguous, admitting of a different explanation, it is difficult to speak correctly on the subject. At Vourla, in Asia Minor, and in some parts of Greece, we found several cases of marsh fever at a considerable elevation above the level of the sea, particularly on the sides of hills planted (though not thickly) with wood ; but, as small patches of land only could be cultivated on these ridges, the inhabitants who live on the higher grounds, like all other persons similarly placed, are forced to seek their subsistence in the low, flat neighbouring country. Cultiva-

* Dr. Hennen's Medical Topography, page 33.

E

tion of the soil in these countries is much in the hands of the
women, and, as the men are too indolent to take the management even of the children in their absence, the poor females
have no other resource left them but to carry their children to
the place where they toil from morning till night. Whole
groups of people, chiefly women and children, are seen collected in different parts of the plains and valleys. Sometimes
a temporary shed is erected, by driving four posts into the
ground, and making a roof with the branches of trees. On
a floor of this kind raised about five feet from the ground,
they rest, and sometimes sleep all night. On these accounts
the women and children are frequently sufferers from marsh
fever. In one instance, we attended a mother and four of
her children, all labouring under the disease, while the hus-
band, a stout brawney Turk, remained in perfect health.
Here then we are furnished with an explanation—why in the
higher grounds marsh fever may prevail, while the inhabitants of the lower are little affected, for the former being
accustomed to breathe the purer air of their native hills,
cannot fail of being more susceptible of marsh effluvia, when
suddenly exposed to their influence. The observation made
by Dr. Johnson, in the passage last quoted from his work, is
so far correct.—Where he says the inhabitants of elevated
districts may be as severely affected with miasmata as if
they were derived from their original source, he seems to be
incorrect; but where he adds, " especially when the predisposing causes are in great force," he is right; but what he
here calls the predisposing causes, *which require to be in
great force*, we would term miasmata, derived from their
original and usual source, namely, the low grounds.

2nd. *Marsh Miasmata become innocuous at a short distance from their source.*

The above instances serve to˘ shew how much marsh
effluvia are restricted in their operation upwards. Their
limited operation in other directions is equally well ascer-

tained; but, as this is a matter of much consequence, we think it necessary to quote proofs from some of the best authors.

In the year 1747, the epidemic marsh fever raged in Zealand, both among the inhabitants and the British troops; and Sir John Pringle says, that Commodore Mitchell's squadron, which lay; all this time at anchor in the channel, between South Beveland and the Island of Walcheren, at both which places the epidemic prevailed, was neither affected with the fever nor flux, but amidst all that sickness enjoyed perfect health.—*Diseases of the Army*, p. 57.

The whole width of the channel is, as Dr. Bancroft believes, in general, but little more than one mile, and therefore the squadron could not, even at midway, be placed at more than half that distance from the grounds whence noxious miasmata arose. Dr. Lind, on preserving the health of seamen, page 69, notices this fact, and makes the following addition to it, viz : When Commodore Long's squadron, in the months of July and August, 1744, lay off the mouth of the Tiber, it was observed that one or two of the ships which lay nearest the shore, began to be affected by the pernicious vapour from the land; whilst some others, lying further out at sea, at but a very small distance from the former, had not a man sick at the same time. The Austrian army, under the command of Prince Lobcowitz, suffered so great a sickness, through the proximity of their situation to the marshy country, that they were obliged to decamp.

Dr. Blane, in his book on the health of seamen, says, "there is reason to believe that marsh miasmata extends to a very small distance." When ships anchored at Rock-fort, Jamaica, says he, "they found that if they anchored close to the shore, so as to smell the land air, the health of the men was affected, but upon removing two cables length, no inconvenience was perceived."—P. 206.

On the late expedition to Zealand, Drs. Blane, Lampriere,

&c., in their report to the Secretary of war, dated Middle-
burg, October 16, 1809, and printed by order of the House
of Commons, assert their having ascertained that the crews
of the vessels stationed in the very narrow channel (only a
few yards from the island), between Beveland and Walcheren, have continued perfectly healthy the whole campaign;
thus decidedly proving that the noxious exhalation is nearly
confined to its own original source. Here it should be
recollected, that it is stated in the same report, that the
number of sick and convalescent in the different hospitals,
amounted to more than two-thirds of the total force at that
time, notwithstanding about 1,500 sick had been already
sent home by different conveyances from Walcheren alone.
The ships of war and transports were generally healthy.
Captain Hanchett, who commanded the Raven sloop of war
during the expedition against Zealand, being wounded, he
remained thirteen nights in shore for the cure of his wounds,
by which he contracted an obstinate intermittent. In his
letter dated Exeter, 27th April, 1810, Captain H. writes as
follows :—" The Raven, when I commanded her on the late
expedition, was more through the narrow channels of Zealand, and more in shore than any other vessel of any description employed there; her station being that of the leading ship of the squadron in shore withal : and, after the
action of the third of August, I went up the narrow passage
between Schowen and Goree (within four miles of William-
stadt), laying not more than a pistol shot from that shore,
and was the last down upon the retreat. There was, however, no ague in the ship but mine, which was no doubt
occasioned by my wound; and, I believe, there were very
few in the other vessels of Commodore Owen's squadron." It
is needless to accumulate proof of a fact so universally established and generally admitted as the narrow sphere of
the operation of marsh poison. Lancisi, Baglivi, and every
author from their time, have furnished us with most convincing proofs of this fact.

3rd. Marsh Miasmata are most concentrated near the earth's surface in the evenings and mornings.

That marsh miasmata are more injurious during the night is a fact equally well known. This greater noxious power to the night, and especially during sleep, has been strongly asserted by Lancisi.—*(De Noxiis Paludum Effluviis, p. 77,* &c.)—He has devoted a particular chapter, the 21st, to explain the cause. " Cur juxtu puludes noctu præsertim indormientes magis quam vigilantes lædantur." And he begins this chapter by saying :—" Nemo arbitror de facti veritate dubitabit qui diu medicæ arte operam dederit." Baglivi confirms the observations of Lancisi on the subject; and, in fact, it has been so long understood at Rome, that travellers proceeding through the Pontine Marshes, which requires only six or eight hours travelling, have always been advised to avoid doing so at night. All books of travels or tours through Italy contain directions of this kind, and the shepherds take refuge in Rome during the night, with a view to avoid their well-known bad effects. It does not seem to be difficult to account for it, as the marsh effluvia is much more condensed near the surface of the earth, and the bodies of those exposed to them are rendered more susceptible to their influence, by the fatigues of the previous day ; in this way Lancisi explains the fact. May not the absence of light also partly account for it ? we know that the power of digitalis and other narcotic poisons is destroyed by light, which in some instances seems to have a specific influence on dead as on living plants, however different its effects may be in these two instances. Dr. John Buon, who practised formerly at Rome, and who we met at Algiers, a short time before the arrival there of the late French expedition, is of opinion, that even the artificial light of lamps will completely prevent the bad effects of marsh effluvia in the most pestiferous of all atmospheres, that of Rome itself. Unless the rays of light of the sun be separated from the calorific rays, no experiment on this head can be conclusive; because the good effects produced might be owing to the heat rarifying the air of the place, and not to light as a separate agent. Lamps producing smoke and heat at the same time, are still less conclusive evidence of the power of light. The following instance may be given among a thousand others that could be added of their speedy operation in this way:—In a voyage to the coast of Guinea, performed in the year 1766, by the Phœnix ship of war, of 40 guns, the officers and ship's company were perfectly healthy, till, on their return home, they touched at the island of St. Thomas. Here the captain unfortunately went on shore, to spend a few days in a house belonging to the Portuguese Governor of that island; this happened during the rainy or sickly season. In the same house were lodged the captain's brother, the surgeon, some midshipmen, and the captain's servant. But in a few days after their being on shore, the captain, his brother, the surgeon, and every one, to the number of seven, who had slept in that house were taken ill, and all of them died except one, who returned to England in a very weak state of health. The ship lay at anchor there twenty-seven days, during which time three midshipmen, five men and a boy, remained on shore for twelve nights, to guard the water-casks, under pretence that the islanders would steal them, all of whom were likewise taken ill, and two of them only escaped with life.

In the late memorable expedition to Java, several men of war were sent to cruize along the coast for several months, before the arrival of the rest of the expedition. During this interval, some flags of truce were sent to Batavia, with dispatches to Governor Dundaels. It was remarked by our officers, that the governor on these occasions was extremely polite, and seldom omitted asking the officers and men to remain with him during the night. This, however, was always avoided, as the motives of the governor were more than suspected, it being well known that such an experiment in such a climate would prove fatal to most of the boat's crew.

CHEMICAL PROPERTIES.—We have no experiments on the nature of marsh poison which are at all satisfactory, but those of White and Seybert (*see the Philosophical Transactions, No.* 9, *p.* 49) seem to support the doctrines laid down as far as they go. Blackburn, in his work on the Prevention of Scarlet Fever, gives the following account of these experiments.

The following, says he, may be considered a very satisfactory confirmation of the doctrine, that pyrexial gases arise from mud in any situation, as well as that of marshes. That they are pyrexial gases chemically constituted, and that they cannot exist under certain attractions of caloric and water is exhibited in the experiments of Dr. White and Dr. Seybert. These experiments were totally unknown to me previously to the conclusions which I had formed from the foregoing facts now quoted, from which they were drawn. I shall present my readers with such extracts from these experiments as are relevant to our subject.

I am of opinion, says Dr. Seybert, that the hydrogen gas is afforded by the decomposition of the stagnant water, effected by the putrefaction of the dead animal and vegetable substances, which enter largely into the composition of the soil of marshes. I was induced to form this opinion, because, first, pure water is a compound of but two elements, consequently, the affinity cannot be broken but by the action of a third substance ; and secondly, we have no experiments to prove that pure water has undergone spontaneous decomposition. My ideas are confirmed by a fact known to all seamen, viz. when a candle is applied to a bung-hole of a cask containing river water, which had been for some time closely stopped, an elastic fluid escapes which will inflame,

and appears in all respects similar to hydrogen gas obtained
by other means.

After forming the above conjectures, I determined to per-
form a few experiments, which might tend to confirm or dis-
prove my opinions. With this view, mud and water, with a
very small portion of atmospheric air, were at different times
closely confined in bottles, closely stopped and inverted over
water. In some instances, the experiment was continued
during twenty and thirty days. They were subjected to the
temperature of the atmosphere. During the progress of the
experiments, I perceived that an elastic fluid was disengaged
from the materials contained in the bottles, and that the water
was certainly diminished in bulk. The elastic fluid generated
during these experiments, 1st, instantly formed a copious
white precipitate when agitated with lime water; secondly,
it burned when the flame of a candle was applied to it, and
possessed the other properties which are common to air obtained by agitating stagnant water over marshes. The above
experiments teach us that mud vitiates the atmosphere in a
very powerful manner. They also enable us to account for
the presence of elastic fluid forming the atmosphere of
marshes. It appears that the carbon of the mud unites
with the oxygen of the decomposed water, and forms the carbonic acid gas, whilst the hydrogen gas is set at liberty.
These are truths not to be invalidated by gratuitous assertions,
since there is experiment. That the atmosphere of marshes
therefore differs in certain circumstances from that of other
situations, and that the soil has considerable effect in altering
the air of the atmosphere, I think, cannot be doubted. Let
us, therefore, endeavour to discover the particular local
causes which give rise to these variations. I have, therefore, hinted, that the putrefaction of animal and vegetable
matters upon the soil of marshes, was the great cause of the
changes observed to exist; for every species of soil will not
operate in the manner alluded to. *That the cause is in the
putrefaction of these matters,* and that this state is absolutely

necessary to those changes, I infer from the following circumstances. Marshes have no noxious influence *during the winter season*. They cause disease when the circumstances are present *which promote putrefaction*, as a proper degree of heat, a due quantity of moisture, and the contact of atmospheric air ; or substances capable of affording oxygen, as water. That a certain degree of moisture is necessary appears evident from White's experiments related in the Philosophical Transactions. He says a certain degree of moisture seems necessary to produce the bad effects of marshes, for mud *when perfectly dry* did not alter the air. He might have added, that too much fluidity will likewise prevent their bad consequences, which is proved by the neighbourhood being healthy when overflowed. An overflow of water may operate by preventing the powerful effects of the sun. Experience teaches us, that their bad effects are discontinued when they *become dry*. Covering them with clay, and other substances *not liable to putrefaction, destroys their bad effects*, and so does cultivation, frost, &c. Living trees being planted in their neighbourhood renders the situation more healthy, by absorbing the gas exhaled during putrefaction and affording oxygen gas. White's experiments prove, first, during sixteen hours, air confined in a phial over water did not suffer change; secondly, fine clay moistened did not alter the purity of the air; thirdly, land moistened did not alter the purity of the air ; but, fourthly, mud (which consists of earths intimately mixed with dead animal and vegetable substances) rendered the air very impure, as I proved by the experiments which I performed.

M. Julia has sixty times subjected to trial the air of different marshes, particularly those on the coast of Cotte, to experiment, but without having arrived at any satisfactory result ; azot, carbonic acid gas, hydrogen, carburetted and sulphuretted hydrogen, have all been fixed upon without proof.

We have now noticed the principal circumstances connected with the generation of marsh poison, as also its mechanical and chemical properties. From what has been said, we think the following conclusions may be safely made. 1st. Marsh poison is a product of putrefaction, and is regulated in some respects by similar laws. 2nd. If this poison exist in a place, it will never be long of shewing itself in some shape or other, for even where its existence cannot be at once referred to the locality, still it must be known from its effects. 3d. Marsh poison must exist in all unhealthy places of any extent, in different degrees of concentration. On this account, marsh fevers will never be of one type or form, but must always vary in this respect according to the degree of concentration of the cause. They will therefore be of different forms *at the same time in the same place,* and this quite independent of the age, sex, or constitution of the person exposed.* 4th. The severest form of marsh fever is not likely to occur in one place or province of an extensive country, and leave every other free; because in all provinces or countries similarly placed there must be many localities possessing the required degree of heat, air, rest, moisture, &c. to operate with similar power on the animal and vegetable matters present. Natural causes are regulated by precisely the same laws in every country, in every part of a country, inland as well as commercial, and in all ages alike. 5th. Marsh fevers for a similar reason can never prevail *to the same extent,* or in the *same form,* in any country *throughout the year,* nor for several years together; for we know of no country, or part of a country, where the climate, seasons, or circumstances are not undergoing material changes, some of which must be inimical to putrefaction. 6th. Marsh fevers will prevail *more or less every year* in those places and seasons which are favourable for their production. 7th. As marsh poison exists in a gaseous state and may be diffused in the atmosphere to a considerable extent, *it can never travel contrary to the wind, or from individual to individual,*

---

* We mean to say here that the cause will produce different forms of marsh fever, as well as the age, sex, or constitution of the patient.

in a slow or gradual manner, for the three following reasons:
Susceptibility is not confined to persons living in one house,
or in one neighbourhood; nor is it regulated in any way by
intercourse or communication with those labouring under
marsh fever; nor is there any mode by which the surrounding atmosphere may be breathed by some individuals and
avoided by others equally exposed. Lastly. The modern
doctrine of the omnipresence of marsh poison to a hurtful
degree is contradicted by fact, by reason, and analogy.

If our view of the subject (marsh miasmata) be correct, it
seems very evident that, wherever these effluvia are applied
to the purposes for which Nature intended them, viz. to
diseases known and universally acknowledged to be of marsh
origin, an explanation of the different phenomena connected
with their history is easy, on the principles of putrefaction.
On the contrary, whenever an attempt is made to extend
their influence beyond its proper bounds, and to put them
down as the essential cause of yellow fever, typhus, plague,
tooth-ache, &c. &c. &c., the thread of connexion between
them and putrefaction is instantly lost. Doctors Bancroft,
Ferguson, and Jackson, stand at the head of the list of non-
contagionists in yellow fever. Of the three, Doctor B. has
the most merit in this, that in spite of all the difficulties
into which his theory has involved him, still he remains
stanch to known philosophical principles. So far as he traces
the connexion between animal and vegetable decomposition
and the different forms of marsh fever, his work is one of the
highest order. When he goes beyond this boundary, he finds
that marsh fevers prevail to a great extent in marshy situations, varying in severity from the mildest intermittent to the
worst form of remittent, *where no cases of yellow fever ever
appear.* He again finds yellow fever in its most frightful
form *without the mildest and intermediate forms,* nay, where
the latter *are scarcely known.* He blames vegetables where
none are present; marshes, where none can be seen; moisture, on a dry rocky soil; high temperature, although the

heat be twenty degrees lower than in neighbouring countries;
certain seasons, though the disease rage in a place *throughout the year, or even for several years together ;* unhealthy
locality, though, like Barbadoes, Cadiz and Gibraltar, they
be places noted for their salubrity. Yellow fever disappears
from the face of the whole globe *for nearly half a century,*
and then starts up in a *single place only,* in spite of the
animal and vegetable decomposition that is going on *in all
ages* and *in different countries ;* still he remains true to his
point, that marsh miasmata is the cause of yellow fever, and
that these effluvia are only produced by animal and vegetable
decomposition.

Dr. Ferguson's creed is somewhat different. He believes
miasmata and malaria* to be the cause of yellow fever ; but,
aware of the difficulties of Dr. Bancroft, he tries to overturn
the generally received opinion of aqueous and vegetable decomposition, singly or combined, being the cause of these
effluvia, and he denies that putrefaction in any shape has the
smallest share in producing them. With the view of supporting his theory, the Doctor has eagerly laid hold of a few
apparent anomalies in the history of marsh fever. We have
already noticed one of these, namely, the occurrence of this
disease on hills and mountains, at a considerable elevation
above the level of the sea or the surrounding country; but
this circumstance, as we have before shown, can be explained
on ordinary principles. He contends that malaria never
emanates from water in bulk, however putrid; but is a product of the highly advanced stage of the drying process, in

* By the term malaria, Dr. Ferguson means to express something
which never belongs to open marshes, but a product of under-ground
moisture, a more subtle miasm which can only be sublimed so as to produce its specific effects on the human body by long continued solar heat.
The terms marsh poison, miasmata, effluvia, exhalation, are meant by
us to express the same thing. In some places we have applied the word
element to the atmosphere, to water and to caloric, as being a moie
popular term.

absorbent soils that had previously and recently been saturated with water. Besides its attraction for lofty umbrageous
trees and rising grounds in the neighbourhood of swamps, he
notices its concentration in ravines and hollows, its absorption by passing over water, its rarefaction or dissolution by
the sun's heat and by regular currents of wind.—Vide *Trans.
of the Royal Society of Edinburgh.*

We have devoted another part of the work to the consideration of miasmata as the cause of yellow fever; and shall,
therefore, not enter at length into an examination of Dr.
Ferguson's opinions here. It may be remarked, however,
that, if malaria be "the product of a highly advanced stage
of the drying process in absorbent soils that had previously
and recently been saturated with water," frequent and heavy
rains could never render marsh fevers prevalent in so many
countries as Dr. Bancroft has pointed out (Vide *Essay*,
p. 199) ; nor could the first rains prove injurious, as Dr.
Johnson and other respectable writers have demonstrated.
In such instances, it is not the drying but the wetting process that proves injurious to health in exciting marsh fever.

Dr. Jackson takes a still greater latitude of opinion than
either Dr. Bancroft or Dr. Ferguson ; he adheres to known
principles so far as they will go in explaining yellow fever,
but adopts others without scruple whenever it is convenient
to call them into play. According to him, chemical mutations in the structural constituents of the earth, or mechanical alterations in its organic adjustments, frequently produce
changes in the atmosphere, and affect its salubrity in such a
manner as to prove a cause of marsh and yellow fever. The
utter impossibility of explaining any of the known properties of the atmosphere on the principle of chemical and
mechanical mutations in the ingredients composing the
earth, has already been pointed out under the head Natural
History of the Atmosphere. The unwieldy materials here
pressed into the service by Dr. J. are as remarkable for being
unsusceptible of chemical change, even when subjected to

the action of the most powerful chemical agents, as they are for being immoveably fixed to the positions allotted for them, probably from the creation of the world itself : none of them possess the power of locomotion. We know of no agent that exists in the bowels of the earth that can impart to them this miraculous quality; and the earth itself is known to be a bad conductor even of caloric. Bodies so little susceptible of chemical change themselves, are not likely to operate in effecting those changes upon others, even under the most favourable circumstances, far less without being brought into close contact with each other, without being reduced to powder by the hammer, without being dissolved by fire or water, or in fact operated upon by any other agent, either to assist the decomposition of the old materials or promote the formation of the new. 2nd. Chemical mutations in the structural constituents of the earth cannot account for marsh and yellow fever. Those diseases prevail most in *hot climates* at *certain seasons* of the year; but there is no difference either in the structural constituents or organic adjustments to explain this fact. They are known to be the same in hot climates as they are in a thousand places where marsh and yellow fever are unknown ; nor is there any thing in climate or season which can possibly operate in effecting a change, except alternations of temperature. But an increase of 20 or 30 degrees of heat is not likely to penetrate deep enough ; far less is it likely that the earth should be a bad conductor of caloric throughout the world generally, yet become a good conductor in certain places at certain seasons. Again, if it be contended that the volcanic, not the sun's heat operates, the same difficulties arise, for we know of no connexion that exists between volcanic changes and climate or season ; those who believe in this are at once brought back to the days of Noah Webster, and to doctrines probably as ancient as the antediluvian Noah himself. Dr. Hunter, in his book on the Diseases of the Army in Jamaica, p. 283, says, "We may, I think, from all the observations we

are yet in possession of, conclude that there is at present no
source of heat in the earth capable of affecting the temperature of a country which is not derived from the sun;
and the earth, whatever changes of temperature it may be
conjectured to have undergone in former periods, is now
reduced to a mean of the heat produced by the sun in different seasons and in different climates." Dr. Nooth found
the water in the wells at New-York, which are from 32 to
40 feet deep, to have an annual variation of temperature of
two degrees only, viz. from 54 to 56. 3rd. According to
those who support this doctrine, both marsh and yellow
fevers have frequently broken out in ships at sea, where
structural constituents of the earth were still less likely to
have any effect. Lastly, marsh fevers have been removed
from whole countries by cultivation of the soil, and other
things incapable of producing chemical or mechanical mutations in the deeper organic constituents and adjustments.

With regard to the ubiquity of marsh poison, a doctrine which can scarcely be treated seriously, opinions
have been advanced still more extraordinary than those
we have just examined. According to some of the writers
who advocate the doctrine of non-contagion in yellow
fever in the American Medical Repository, a few bags of
rotten potatoes or apples may excite yellow fever in a place,
yet many millions of acres of putrefying animal and vegetable matters be insufficient. It is in fact impossible to read
all the arguments, contentions and bickerings, contained in
its volumes on this head, without suspecting that marsh
poison exerts its peculiar powers on those who study it,
as well as on those who have been really exposed to its
noxious influence. As some writers see every thing through
a mist of marsh miasmata, imperfect vision becomes of
course the pathognomonic symptom of their disease. Some
things seem large in the fog, while others are totally obscured; distorted objects become straight, and straight ones
become distorted ; the jaundiced eye succeeds, and the

paroxym often terminates in spleen and bad humour. Whether on a *post-mortem* examination, the spleen or the encephalon would be found in the state of cake* remain to be proven.

To those who believe that the Turkey carpet of the parlour, or the marble table of the lobby, may occasionally generate marsh poison, some of their arguments may prove convincing. On the other hand, those who consider attentively the principles before explained, that putrefaction, like every other important process of Nature, is regulated by fixed laws and restrained within certain bounds; that its products are not allowed to accumulate, so as to corrupt air and water under ordinary circumstances; that a number of agents must act simultaneously on dead organised matter for a certain time and in due proportions, before these noxious effluvia can be generated or let loose; that dead organised matter never abounds in all places alike, or even in a considerable number at the same time; that what is favourable for its decomposition in one locality is unfavourable in others; that, in most places where decomposition does take place, living vegetables and other counteracting causes are in perpetual operation to prevent its bad effects on animal or vegetable life; lastly, that the sphere of action of marsh poison itself is very limited, both in a horizontal and perpendicular direction; we say, those who consider these things, must be inclined to pause before they admit either the validity of the doctrines or the soundness of the arguments set forth in their support. In short, we can see no reason to abandon the old and established theory of animal and vegetable decomposition being the cause of marsh fever, except the one too often used by the mere dogmatic, that it is a vulgar belief, and a doctrine too easily brought down to the level of the common understanding.

---

* The morbid enlargement of the spleen, so often observed in those who have died of marsh fevers, is called ague cake.

The effects of marsh miasmata on the human system next fall to be considered. We shall notice those chiefly *which serve to point out the mode of prevention ;* as the time they remain latent in the system, how they enter the body, the persons most liable to their influence, their mode of action, whether or not they affect the same person repeatedly, the consequences of long exposure, &c. &c. The lungs and stomach are probably the only channels by which they can enter the body. " When we consider," says Dr. Johnson, " that, at each inspiration, the atmosphere impregnated with this principle is largely applied to the delicate texture of the lungs, it is not difficult to conceive, that it may pass into the blood (if it is in any case absorbed) as readily as oxygen. There are, besides, the Schneiderian, and other membranes of the nares and fauces, to which it must have constant access, while there is but one way for it to pass into the stomach, viz. along with the saliva or food. Further, when we see this principle, in a concentrated state, produce fever *in a very few hours,* with high delirium, can we suppose that it enters the system by the circuitous route of the alimentary canal and lacteals ? If it be said that it acts through the medium of the nerves of the stomach, why not through that of the olfactory, which is a shorter road ? Indeed, from a near view of its *effects,* there is every reason to suppose that the brain and nervous system suffer the first impression and shock."

The time these effluvia take in producing their known effects is different, according to circumstances. Dr. Johnson mentions a very few hours as being sufficient to produce fever with high delirium, where the principle is in a concentrated state. According to him, also, the latent period varies from one day to eighteen, twenty, or even thirty days, according to the degree of concentration, and even then brings on fever only in consequence of some of the predisposing or auxiliary causes concurring to enable the original to develop itself; but the ordinary period is twelve or fourteen days. Doctor Jackson extends the latent period to two months. Doctor

F

Hunter says, "though he had reason to suspect that this period might be much greater than three weeks, he had not any facts or observations that were decisive on the subject ; but, in 1793, the West Suffolk regiment of Militia, after suffering from marsh fever so severely at Hilsea Barracks that they lost twenty-two men between the months of February and the latter end of June, encamped in the first week of July at Waterdown, in the neighbourhood of Tunbridge Wells. From the fatigues of the march and the duties of the camp, their sick list soon amounted to one hundred out of five hundred, and of these there were thirty ill of fevers in the hospital, which had all the characteristic marks of a bad remittent. During the four months of the campaign, there died of fevers in this regiment twelve, a greater number than what died of all other diseases put together in the eleven other battalions that were encamped on the same ground ; and, in the month of October, some were taken ill of the fever who had never had it before, that is nearly four months after they had ceased to be exposed to the cause of the disease at Hilsea Barracks."—Vide pp. 330-1.

If the men last mentioned by Dr. H. had not been exposed to marsh effluvia at Waterdown or its neighbourhood in the interval, this must be regarded as proof of the latent period being extended sometimes to four months ; but, for our part, we strongly suspect that they were so exposed during their campaign. The name Waterdown gives grounds for this suspicion ; and we think it probable, that the men of the West Suffolk Militia, encamping during the hot months and after their fatigue from their increased duty, owing to the sickness of so great a proportion of the men of the regiment, might suffer from the marsh effluvia of the place, when those belonging to the other battalions remained tolerably healthy. "From comparing," says Dr. Lind, "many instances of people who have slept on shore during the sickly season, and, in consequence of it, who *alone have been taken ill out of the whole ship's company* then lying in an open road, it appears that some are *immediately* seized with sickness or delirium; many are not seized with either till they have been on board *two or three days ;* several have been only slightly indisposed for the first five or six days ; and in a *few,* the symptoms of indisposition have not appeared before *the tenth or twelfth day."—On Climate,* p. 182. The same author says, in his book on the Health of Seamen, p. 78, " I have known *the whole of a boat's crew seized next morning* with bad fevers," that is after sleeping near the mangroves with which the sides of rivers are frequently planted in the Torrid Zone.

But such very sudden attacks of fever from marsh effluvia, Doctor Bancroft thinks are uncommon, even in the hottest climates or worst situations. They, indeed, occur *not unfrequently* within four or five days, but are much oftener delayed until the ninth, twelfth, and fifteenth days, after exposure to marsh miasmata, even at Batavia, Gambia, St. Thomas, Mohilla, &c. Dr. Jackson, who, like some others, is disposed to believe that these attacks take place chiefly at septenary periods, asserts, from his own observation made on numerous bodies of men and upon healthy soldiers sent to the concentrated sources of endemic fever, that, among such, fever scarcely ever appeared before the *seventh,* commonly not before the *fourteenth,* and in numerous instances not till the expiration of *six weeks or two months,* though the cause of the disease during that time was ordinarily in great activity.—*Outline, &c. of Fever,* p. 248—*Bancroft,* p. 238.

After this passage, Dr. B. quotes the instance of the West Suffolk Militia, noticed above, along with that of the 18th regiment of Foot in 1783-4, given on the authority of Mr. Venour, then surgeon of the regiment ; also from Dr. Hunter's work, and proceeds to state " that *considerable numbers,* both of officers and soldiers, who escaped the sickness whilst at Walcheren and other parts of Zealand, were attacked by intermitting fevers ; and *some of them* as late as *six, seven, eight,* and even *nine months* after being brought back to this country, though care was taken to place them generally in situations remote from all the known sources of marsh miasmata." From this, the Doctor thinks " that *vernal* intermittents may now be considered as resulting from marsh miasmata received into the body during the preceding Summer or Autumn, and, after having remained in a quiescent state during Winter, rendered active by some exciting or proximate cause of fever in the Spring. It may be presumed, however, that, in such cases, the original dose, if I may so call it, was but moderate, because its effects would otherwise have been sooner manifested; and this will account for the well known mildness of vernal intermittents, and the facility with which they are generally cured."—*Essay, p.* 242.

We are sorry to be obliged so often to criticise the statements and opinions of Dr. Bancroft, but the conclusion he draws here is too important to be rested on such premises. The original dose of the poison, to the influence of which the soldiers had been exposed at Walcheren and other parts of the island of Zealand before their return to England, could not be so very moderate as only to be able to excite marsh fever of the mildest and most easily cured form, and that at a long interval of nine months, as he supposes and takes for granted, when it is considered that, out of 1738 officers and 37,481 rank and file, who sailed from England in July, 1809, 217 officers and 11,296 rank and file returned home sick in September of the same year. The number that died in Zealand is not taken into the account here; but Sir James Fellowes, from whose reports we have taken this statement, says, " taking the full number of admissions into the different hospitals (in England) at 17,536 and the deaths at 914, the proportion will therefore only be one in nineteen; but if we deduct about *four thousand* from the general return as supposed re-admitted cases, or relapses, and patients transferred from the different hospitals, then the proportion of deaths will be nearly one in fifteen.—*Reports, p.* 390. So much for the moderate dose of the poison on which Dr. B's theory is founded, and that dose which can only excite *mild* and *easily cured* intermittents. The above returns only include the ad - missions and deaths in England between the month of September, 1809, and the 1st of February, 1810; but at the last period, when marsh poison ought to have been asleep and those who had suffered from its effects recovered, 2327 sick still remained in the hospitals at Colchester, Harwich, Norwich, Yarmouth, Ipswich, and Woodbridge, to which places the army went on its return from Zealand. Might not " *some* of the considerable number" of men who remained free from intermittent fevers, six, seven, eight, and even nine months after their return to England, be exposed to marsh poison in any of the above towns or their neighbourhoods in the intervals? Those who were six months exempted would take ill in March, the others in April, May and June, when marsh poison in England would be sufficiently powerful to excite a mild intermittent in persons predisposed to the disease. Colchester, Harwich, and Woodbridge, are all in the county of Essex, one of the fenny districts of England; and Norwich and Yarmouth are near Lincolnshire, another of the same kind, so that the soldiers had not a great way to walk before coming within the sphere of marsh effluvia.

While Dr. B. questions the possibility of marsh poison being generated in such parts of England in the months of March, April, May, and June, sufficiently powerful to excite the mildest form of marsh fever, Dr. O'Halloran, another miasmatic and noncontagionist in yellow fever, and an author on the Epidemic of Barcelona in 1821, brings forward no less than fifteen Spanish physicians who had signed a manifesto against contagion, to assert that " fevers attended with black vomit, yellowness, &c. (in other words marsh fevers of the worst form according to the noncontagionists) annually appear in the city of Barcelona and in Barcelonetta, in the months of February, March, April, May, and June."—P. 28. Still Dr. O'Halloran is not quite pleased with the Spanish

physicians for not coming sufficiently fast over to the miasmatic side, but sagely remarks—"The dismission of prejudice is not the work of a day. Would the Spaniards
permit themselves to draw conclusions from an accurate
knowledge of the general laws of the epidemics of the Mediterranean coast of Spain," &c. If the heat on the continent of
Europe be sufficient to generate and separate miasmata strong
enough to excite fevers attended with black vomit, yellowness,
&c. every year in February, will not the temperature of the
month of June in England be sufficient to produce the mildest
and most easily cured intermittent ? By such vague theories
only can the more generally received doctrines regarding
marsh poison be assailed, and the time it remains latent in
the system has often led to a belief that it exists in places
where there are no apparent causes from which its existence
might be inferred. Thus, those persons who have been accustomed to breathe a pure air, are from that very circumstance more susceptible ; and it has been said that some of
the inhabitants of fenny districts occasionally turn it to their
own profit, by choosing one rich help-mate as another dies,
from the higher and dryer parts of the country, a proof, at
least, of the fact being pretty generally known.

On the same principle, strangers are most liable to be
affected with marsh poison. The countrymen who come down
in the harvest time into the Campagna Modina, Ferrara,
Bresse, &c. where the rice grounds and marshy districts are
principally situated, are most frequently attacked with the
fever, even when the season is considered favourable by the
natives. A similar observation was made at Walcheren. It
was also remarked, that strangers were variously affected,
according to the district whence they came. Thus it was
found, that those of the British troops who were natives of
mountainous districts and dry soils, were more frequently
affected than the natives of flat and moist counties.

It was ascertained by General Monet, who commanded the
French troops in Flushing during the whole of the seven years

in which it was in their possession, that the troops should not be frequently changed, for when it was the custom to send battalions from Bergen-op-Zoom every fourth night in succession to work on the lines of Flushing, these men never failed to be taken ill in great numbers. General Monet, therefore, advised that a stationary garrison should be retained in Walcheren, in order that it might be habituated to the air (acclimate), and he adduced an instance in his memoir, which he left behind him after the capture of the island, of a French regiment which suffered only one half the sickness and mortality in the second year of its being there, that it experienced during the first half year, and it scarcely suffered at all in the third.* Persons lose this insusceptibility to marsh effluvia by removing to and living some time in places where the air is dry and more pure. Even the inhabitants of one marshy district become susceptible on removing to another marshy place. In general, it will be found that sailors, accustomed to breathe the pure air of the ocean, are more liable to be affected on that account, but particularly if they remove from a cold to a warmer latitude. If persons are exposed to the exhalations of marshes when fatigued with hard labour and long fasting, the poison gains admission more readily into the body, and produces immediately the worst kind of fever. But although this fact, and the danger of being exposed to the air of marshes in the evenings when the effluvia become concentrated near the earth's surface, and in the mornings before the power of the sun is sufficient to dissipate them, have been long known, yet, no sooner had the British troops reached their notoriously marshy destination *in the most unhealthy season* of the year 1809, than these *strangers* to Zealand were ordered *to be under arms every morning an hour before day-light*. From this short sentence then, it appears that every known principle of marsh effluvia was set at nought. The young and robust are parti-

* Vide Quarterly Review, Vol. xxviii.

cularly liable to marsh fever as to plague, and partly from the same causes, that being less careful of themselves, they are of course more exposed to the poisons, as well as to the different exciting causes. On these accounts, women are not so often attacked as men. Persons having once had marsh fever, are rendered more susceptible. Hence, slight inter-mittents sometimes occur in such persons on board of ships at sea, when all the rest of the crew remain in health, showing that a cause will excite fever in them, which proves inade-quate to excite it in others. We have seen men so affected more than twelve months after they had been exposed to land influence of any kind. Those persons who remain in the same place after their first attack, sometimes become less susceptible from the habit of breathing the same air as before noticed.

The differences in the mode of action of marsh and morbid poisons, will be fully pointed out after the reader has been made acquainted with the laws of contagion. These will be illustrated in our review of the evidence on the nature of yellow fever. The mode of prevention will also be fully noticed in its proper place.

END OF FOURTH DISSERTATION.

PART II.

DISSERTATIONS ON HEALTH.

DISSERTATION V.

OF STATISTICAL CAUSES.

CONTAGION.

AUTHORS have applied different meanings to the terms contagion and infection; some restricting the former to those diseases communicated by contact, and the latter to those capable of being propagated to a short distance from their source, through the medium of the atmosphere. This distinction is objectionable, in so far as it leads to a belief in the existence of two agents instead of one : in both instances the agent is the same, the effects produced upon the subject exposed are the same ; the sphere or power of action of the agent only differs. As chemists, therefore, apply the term heat to the sensation produced by the presence of caloric, instead of applying it to the matter of heat, or the agent itself, so we would use the word infection, to express the existence of contagion in any body. In this view it would be correct to say that a man, a lancet, or a piece of cloth, is infected by contagion, in the same way we say a body is heated by caloric.

We think it right to be explicit in the meaning of terms, as much confusion has arisen from their loose application. Fracastorius and Dr. Charles M'Lean restrict the term contagion to those diseases which occur in the same individual but once during life.

The history of contagion is involved in much obscurity; for although it is occasionally mentioned in the writings of the ancient physicians, philosophers, and even poets, yet no notice is taken of any diseases which occurred but once during life.* A few modern writers have indeed laboured hard to prove the antiquity of small-pox, measles, hooping-cough, venereal disease, &c.; but it seems evident that, had those diseases prevailed to the same extent among the ancient Greeks and Romans as they have done in modern times, no room could possibly have been left for conjecture.

Their medical authors, who have given the most minute description of diseases, far more obscure, and therefore less easily described, were not likely to overlook those of a more prominent character; and, had they existed, their poets would have mourned the loss of beauty, to say nothing of the loss of life and health they occasioned, while the superstitious fears of the people would have created gods and goddesses to preside over their fate, and to protect them in times of danger.

It is not necessary to go so far back in history to prove that little was really known of the nature of contagion. Human effluvia were wholly overlooked in the time of Sydenham, Mead, Huxham, and Short, although every year of their lives must have furnished examples of their dreadful effects on the public health. In an age when physicians were taught to search for the causes of disease in other worlds, not in this; when they contemplated the stars rather than the streets; and when they believed that the atmosphere in which they lived, moved, and had their being, was created more for the destruction than support of animal life; it is not surprising that human effluvia, together with the whole class of statistical causes, should have been entirely overlooked.

---

* It was however remarked, that the plague of Athens never seized the same person twice.

Similar errors prevail to a frightful extent even at the present day. The following passage, taken from the history of the great plague of London, is therefore still applicable.

" Hypochondriac fancies represent,
" Ships, armies, battles in the firmament,
" Till steady eyes the exhalations solve,
" And all to the first matter, cloud, resolve."

Some modern authors seem to have gone into an error of a different kind.

Dr. Adams, one of the most distinguished modern writers, observes, "another circumstance seems necessary to ascertain contagion, namely, that it can only be excited by a cause exactly similar to its effects." Dr. Bancroft, when arguing about the yellow fever which broke out among the settlers at Bulama, in 1792, rejects the idea of any contagious disease being generated on board of ship, or in that Island. He thinks it every way as likely, that the Island of Bulama might produce elephants, without the sexual intercourse of the animals themselves. Now, if we understand the above passages rightly, they point to direct propagation as the only means by which contagion can be produced. According to this view, therefore, the contagions must have been coeval with mankind: they must have descended from generation to generation, like father and son. Abraham must have begat Isaac, Isaac must have begotten Jacob, and so on throughout; although the degrees of relationship and consanguinity must be more difficultly ascertained in the one instance than in the other. If this view be correct, the contagions too must have had an independent existence, and been produced from other sources than man himself: but we are told that our first parents became liable to disease only in consequence of transgression; and in every part of the Holy Scriptures, where any allusions are made to pestilence, it is mentioned as the scourge of cities, and rather as an evil brought on man by sin, than as

originating from a cause over which he had no control, or
with which he had no connexion. What became of the contagions at the universal deluge, supposing them to have been
created at the beginning, we are at a loss to conjecture. The
single family of Noah, unless in a state of disease, were not
likely to hand them down to the post-deluvian world. We
are not told of the different kinds of contagion having been
preserved in the ark like the different species of animals to
be set adrift over the face of the earth, on the subsiding of
the waters; nor does Pagan history inform us of a second
edition of Pandora's box.

As the contagions are now known to be products of diseased, not healthy action of the human system, we cannot believe they were generated at all till man became subject to
those diseases peculiar to certain conditions of society, any
more than we can believe that the poison of the viper existed
before the viper itself. Yet all the contagions must have had a
beginning. If they have once been produced by certain combinations of circumstances, which seems evident, why may
they not again be produced by the same concurrence of causes,
independent of " a cause similar to their effects?" That itch,
scald-head, plica, yaws, syphilis, gonorrhœa, hydrophobia,
typhus fever, and even plague, have all arisen spontaneously
in our own day can scarcely be doubted.

It was formerly believed, that many of the contagions were
natives of Egypt, and that they had travelled from thence over
the rest of the world by different routs. In the earlier ages
of the world it is not probable they existed, or at least prevailed to any extent, owing to the thinner population and er-
ratic habits of mankind. When man was employed in hunt-
ing, fishing, or tending his flocks, the contagions could never
be generated. In proportion, however, as society became
further advanced; when mankind, leaving their primitive
employments in the open air, began to settle in towns, and
engage in arts and commerce, then contagions would extend
and multiply. Egypt and other countries in the East, being

those in which society soonest arrived at the required condition, would undoubtedly also be the first to experience their
baneful effects.

So far then the opinion of their Egyptian origin seems
a correct one, but in any other light it would be every way
as proper to contend that architecture was a native of Egypt,
because this noble art was first brought to great perfection
in that country. Contagion, properly speaking, is confined
to no nation or people. It is not produced by a natural but
artificial state of mankind. Neither the primitive nor most
advanced or civilized condition of society are likely to feel
its effects, but a medium or barbarous one; a state in which
man has attained sufficient knowledge to suit his own worldly
views, without once dreaming of the consequences that must
inevitably follow his gross outrages on the laws of Nature.

No climate, therefore, is of itself sufficient to generate
contagion, without the implied condition.

In the ancient histories of Egypt, according to Assilini, no
mention is made of the plague; and the same author agrees
with Sir John Pringle and Pappon, in thinking that that country was more healthy before it became a province of the Ottoman Empire.

Herodotus assures us that the Egyptians, next to the Ly-
bians, were the most healthy people in existence. He attributes their good constitutions to the constant serenity of the
air, and the unvarying uniformity of the seasons. " When the
plague," says Pappon, " affected the city of Rome, 717 years
before the Christian era, and when it appeared in the reigns
of Numa and Tullus Hostilius, these were the happy days of
Egypt; those of its greatest fertility, of its civilization, culture, and population. Two hundred and fifty years afterwards Egypt had lost none of these advantages. During
the five first centuries pestilence ravaged Italy more than
twenty-five times. In the two last ages of the Republic, to
the end of the reign of Claudius, (or 250 years) it only appeared *three* times on that side of the Alps.

" These were the happy days of Italy, when agriculture and civilization had attained to greatest perfection.

" After the fourth century of the Christian era, Europe was desolated with wars, and pestilence was very frequent; so that from the fifth to the middle of the seventh century, it occurred in the West ten times on an average every hundred years.

" Under the Mussulman's government, Egypt relaxed into that state which has been productive of so many physical and moral evils to its inhabitants."—*De la Peste.*

The exemption of Persia from plague has been noticed by most writers; although their country is every year surrounded by the disease, yet the Persians seldom suffer by it themselves. The Persians are the most cleanly people in the world, and many of them make it part of their religion to remove filth and nuisances of every kind from their persons, cities, and dwellings. They are also favoured by a dry pure air. Boyle has mentioned the exemption of China, on the authority of Alexander de Rhodes, who resided thirty years in that country. Although that empire is so vast and populous, of course possessing every climate supposed to be favourable to plague, it is seldom visited. A country with so many millions of inhabitants, subsisting wholly on vegetables, cannot but be well drained and cultivated.

No fences are to be seen, and scarcely a tree on the plains, lest the husbandman should lose the smallest portion of his ground.* Japan is another country, the exemption of which from pestilence, has also been frequently noticed.—*(See Phil. Trans. Hancock on Pestilence, &c. &c.)*

Besides the cultivation of the soil in China and Japan, the little intercourse their inhabitants have with those of other

* Some few years since a national quarrel was nearly excited between Great Britain and China, by the trivial offence of the crew of a British frigate (we believe the Topaz,) cutting broom in China. In a country where no broom is allowed to grow but what is absolutely required, this was a more serious injury than in most other countries.

nations, and the excellence in many respects of their patriarchal governments, must be taken into view.

The people in both may in fact be said to enjoy most of the advantages of civilization, without feeling many of the evils that arise from epidemic diseases, and which are usually attendant on a great population in other countries.

Lind has taken a fact from Sinæpeus, who says, there are whole nations in Tartary exempted from small-pox. This immunity we have no doubt arises from their wandering habits and mode of life. They do not live in houses, but tents : they spend much of their time in the open air. When they do settle in a small body, they pitch their camps on the driest and most healthy spots only, their tents being kept open at the bottom during the day, so as to admit the free circulation of air; and they never settle long enough in one place to accumulate filth. The wandering tribes of Arabs who observe a similar mode of life, are often known to escape plague at a time when it is raging in a neighbouring town, or even in a camp which has been long settled in the same place. Mexico, according to Humboldt, had never been visited by small-pox before the year 1520; and small-pox, measles, hooping-cough, scarlet fever, &c. are still unknown in New Holland, either to natives or settlers. *(See Cunningham's work on New Holland)*. Till after the Crusades those diseases were but little known in Europe. Plague has not yet reached any part of the New World.

The return of Columbus from America is the date of the first appearance of the venereal disease* in Europe. Sibbens

---

* The South Sea Islanders were free from this disease till the first visits of Europeans spread it amongst them. As no people were more addicted to licentious love, this fact seems to militate against the possibility of its being generated by such indulgence. Where the practice of illicit love is so general amongst both sexes, as to be universal, the danger will be less than where a large proportion of males is confined to a small proportion of the opposite sex. It was such a condition of society which first produced the disease.

is seen in but very few countries. Plica it is said was derived from the Tartars, and now is only to be found amongst the poor in Poland, chiefly amongst the Jews. Hydrophobia is rare in the West Indies; at Malta it is seldom seen. It is unnecessary to multiply facts to show the close connexion that exists between pestilential diseases and certain conditions of society. Volumes might be filled with such facts. Two, however remain, which deserve a place. Before the year 1804, the garrison of Gibraltar had been exempt from yellow fever one hundred years. .Before 1813, Malta had been free from an attack of plague for one hundred and thirty-seven years. Is it at all likely that either place should have enjoyed so long an immunity, had the people been placed under Ottoman laws, or Turkish fanaticism?

At this day a man may spend a long life free from plague in Cairo or Constantinople, if he do not, like Dr. M'Lean, go to the abodes of filth, misery, and wretchedness, to search it out.

What contagious disease is there in our own country that does not follow precisely the same rules?

The following conclusions may be drawn from the history of the contagions :—1st. All of them have been generated without a cause similar to its effects. 2d. That a certain number of concurrent causes, though not sufficient in themselves, may induce that species of unhealthy action in the system which generates them. 3d. The rarity or frequency of their production will depend on the number and nature of the causes required, or the likelihood of their concurrence. 4th. When once produced, they are chiefly maintained by intercourse. Lastly, as none of them are capable of maintaining an independent existence, unless they be preserved in places where they are not exposed to the actions of other agents, it follows that all of them may be destroyed by ventilation, cleanliness, and other means.

The theory of the sanative nature of the acute contagions is contradicted by many facts connected with their history. If, during the occurrence of small-pox, measles, &c. certain matters be thrown out of the system, which, if retained, would injure the constitution, and induce a greater liability to other diseases, it is not easy to comprehend how whole nations which have never had them, should, notwithstanding their exemption, remain in as good health as those who have gone through them ; that is, with the single exception of the latter not being liable to a second attack. The notion, therefore, that there must be a certain quantum of disease, in order to keep down excess of population, is an absurd one. Most of the great cities of Europe are more populous now than they were half a century ago, yet the proportion of deaths in each year from contagious diseases is diminishing, not increasing. This non-liability to a second attack has, perhaps, given rise to the belief of the sanative nature of the contagions. It is one of the most important connected with their history. It serves to account for their prevalence in the same place at distant and uncertain periods. As it restricts their occurrence, it is, without doubt, intended by Nature as a necessary restriction to guard the human race from destruction.

Another thing which accounts for their less frequent occurrence and less general diffusion is, that they are morbid, not natural products of the animal body.

There is no particular organ of the body set apart for the purpose of secreting those poisons during health, as in the case of the viper, and some other venomous animals. But the same organ which is employed for other purposes during health assumes to itself a new creative power during disease. As this is a great effort of the system it does not last long at one time, nor is the body capable of repeating it at a future period. Hence all the acute contagious diseases, which are by far the most violent and dangerous, are necessarily restricted to a few days or weeks in a long life. Death either puts an end to this unnatural process, or the healthy action of the system is resumed.

A third guard against the propagation of the contagions is, that all of them are dependent like plants on soil and climate.

By the term soil, as applied to them, we mean the condition of society.

The human body is not always susceptible. 1st. It may be pre-occupied with some other disease at the time of exposure. As two unhealthy actions are not likely to occur in the same individual at the same time, it often happens that contagion, when applied, is rendered impotent; the one diseased action being inconsistent with the other. If the first morbid condition remain for a length of time, the contagion may be thus destroyed before the person to whom it was applied becomes again liable.

2nd. Certain healthy conditions of the body are unfavourable to the power of contagion. If a healthy person be exposed to contagion, it may happen that his body, at the time of exposure, is rather in an exhaling than absorbing state;— the poison may not be applied a sufficient length of time for absorption taking place, or it may be placed on a part of the surface incapable of absorption.

Much, too, will depend on the dose of the poison; its state of activity; whether it is diffused or concentrated; its purity or mixture with foreign matters, &c. &c. For it is evident that the most virulent of these morbid poisons vary much in their activity according to the time of the disease by which they are produced, to the degree of fever, to the age and sex of the patient from whom they are taken, the violence or mildness of the disease in him or her, and the nature of their constitutions. Besides soil and climate, therefore, the growth of the contagions, like that of plants, must at all times depend *on the quality of the seed.*

But of all the guards placed against the diffusion of contagion the atmosphere is the most powerful. Even in the most favourable state of the air, none of the contagions can operate beyond a few feet or yards from their source. This law of contagion is so important, that we shall afterwards take pains to illustrate it. The state of the atmosphere, with regard to temperature, moisture, dryness, purity, weight, rest, and motion, has such an influence on the contagions, although their effects are not the same in every one, that even good *seed* planted in a tolerable soil may be rendered comparatively unproductive by *season*. Nor is this at all to be wondered at. How often do we see precisely the same thing happen in the vegetable economy, where, in some seasons, all the cares of the farmer or horticulturist will fail in producing a crop with the best seed and soil.

It is probable that contagion can exist in air, either chemically or mechanically, like water or other condition of vapour. It is certainly modified in its activity by the degree of moisture in the atmosphere influencing its solubility. According to Sir Robert Wilson, the English and Turkish armies that marched to Cairo escaped contagion, while the troops that remained stationary on the moist shores of Aboukir were severely visited. Assilini describes the whole surface of Lower Egypt as so much changed, that formerly it might have been the most healthy part of Africa.

The ruins of ancient monuments and cities are in part submersed and surrounded with water. "Of the places which, on account of situation, are protected from the scourge of plague, (says Assilini, p. 59,) the citadel of Cairo is noted as one instance. Its inhabitants, during the plague of 1791, were exempt from the disease which laid waste the lower town, with which, nevertheless, they continued to hold a constant intercourse." "It has been observed, (adds he,) the inhabitants of this fort and environ *have always escaped* from the plague." When the city has been enveloped in a thick mist, he has found the air of the citadel elastic, pure, and light.

The neighbouring countries of Attica and Bœotia in Greece furnished in ancient times a singular confirmation of a similar fact, as mentioned by Webster on the authority of Anacharsis. In Bœotia, where the air was dense, the soil rich and fertile, the country like a bason surrounded with high mountains, having a lake in the centre forty miles in circumference, without an opening into the sea, the people were so frequently visited by plague, as mentioned by Justin, that the Delphic oracle was consulted how the evil was to be removed, and the colonization of Pontus was recommended.

In the neighbouring country of Attica, on the contrary, where the soil is dry and rocky and the air very pure, the inhabitants were seldom visited. Muratori observes " nel ducato di Modena le terre di Vignuola, Guiglia, et tante altre castille della collina, et della montagna quantunque confirmate ad altre infette della pestilenza, o circondata di essa, pure col mezzo delle guardie et delegenza usitata schivarano cosi terribil disaventura."

Alpinus, that " plerumque pestilens, contagium in Egyptum ex multis locis, peste infectis asportari solet; rarissime ab aeris vitio pestis illuc nascitur, *et hoc non nisi, ubi Nilus immodice ea loca inundat.*" Fracastorius, treating of the plague, says " rarissime contigit, ut aeris corruptione pestilentia contingat." The effects of dryness are not less remarkable.

The hermattan, a wind experienced on the western coast of Africa, between the equator and fifteen degrees north latitude, blowing from north-east towards the Atlantic, and which, in consequence of passing over a very extensive space of arid land, is necessarily characterised by excessive dryness, puts an end to all epidemics, as the small-pox, and infection at such a time does not appear to be easily communicated even by art.—*See Philosophical Transactions, Vol. 71.— Paris's Pharmacologia, p. 138.*

In fact the dependence of the contagions on the state of the atmosphere is too well confirmed to require more proof. The fact has been mentioned by most writers, to some of whom it appeared so conspicuous as to mislead them into a belief of its essential agency, both in their generation and after propagation. Hence, both Alpinus and Fracastorius, although they think it was a rare occurrence, nevertheless deem it possible that plague might arise from vitiated or moist air alone.

The marked influence of the atmosphere has been productive of other errors. Some of the contagions (small-pox for one) spread more certainly in different conditions of atmosphere than in others. A contagion like small-pox, possessing the double power of affecting persons by contact or near approach, through the medium of the air, must be less restricted in its propagating power than one which can only operate in one mode. Plague can only be communicated by contact. Typhus and yellow fever are more dependant on the sensible properties of the air than some others. The non-contagionists however, take small-pox as the standard, and some of them contend that plague, typhus, and yellow fever are not contagious, because they do not observe in every instance the exact same law.

It has been well remarked by Professor Hossack, that they might as well reject the belief in contagion of yellow fever, because it was not accompanied with the pustules of small-pox. Every individual of the same species of animal has not the exact same outward form or character; but no one would argue that the fox was not one of the canine tribe, because he possesses more cunning than the dog, or carried a tail of a form somewhat different.

The marked dependence often observed of the contagions on the state of the atmosphere with regard to heat, dryness, moisture, &c. has given rise to a third error, still more unaccountable.

Any one who considers attentively the principles already explained, particularly the number of circumstances, all or most of which must concur, before even contagious diseases can prevail to a great degree, will at once understand why they become epidemical only at distant and uncertain periods. As before said, in proportion to the number of circumstances required, and the likelihood of their concurrence, will be the frequency or rarity of the epidemic attack. When the causes are all present, the disease will prevail in the highest degree, and to the greatest extent. When some of the circumstances are only present, the disease will prevail to a less degree. Where the contagion is present, but both the condition of society and the state of the atmosphere are unfavourable to propagation, the disease will only be partially observed, perhaps not extend beyond the few individuals first affected. It may so happen, however, that the condition of society and the quality of contagion, in other words the soil and seed, may both be so favourable as to produce a good crop or epidemic in seasons where no remarkable changes in the sensible qualities of the air are observable. For example, if the small-pox be introduced into a large populous city, either for the first time, or after a very long interval of immunity from its ravages, few persons will escape an attack of the disease ; whereas, on a second visit, few individuals will be affected by it, unless the generation which has before gone through the disease has died and been succeeded by a new and susceptible race.* The prevalence of a contagious disease, therefore, may depend on the distance of time between two attacks, or on other circumstances totally unconnected with atmospheric influence.

It is true, we cannot always point out the precise nature of those circumstances, no more than we can the causes of the failure of crops in seasons which appeared favourable under similar circumstances of soil and culture. We are yet but imperfectly acquainted with the vegetable as well as the animal economy.

The aerial theorists driven from their ground, namely, the

* " Small Pox," says Humboldt, in his Political Essay on New Spain, " appears only to exercise its ravages in Mexico every seventeen or eighteen years. In equinoxial regions it has, *like the black vomiting* (yellow fever) and several other diseases, its fixed periods, to which it is very regularly subjected. We might say then, in those countries, *the disposition* to certain miasmata *is only renewed in the natives at long intervals.*" This has been observed in other countries as well as Mexico ; the cause of it we have explained.

Humboldt adds that " inoculation and vaccination has lately saved thousands in that country."

essentiality of sensible atmospheric changes for the production of an epidemic, have been forced reluctantly to abandon it, and to confess the utter impossibility of explaining the phenomenon on the principles of the sensible changes of the air. Ever bent, however, to uphold atmospheric omnipotence in some shape or other, they have been led to conjecture, for they can offer no proof, that it arises from some hidden, occult, or unknown qualities existing in the atmosphere. Every thing on the earth beneath, in the waters under the earth, as well as things high in the heavens, have all in their turns been accused.

Hence, the aspect of the stars, the course of the planets, the appearance of comets and meteors, the electric, chemical, and mechanical changes of the air, earthquakes and other convulsions of the earth, its magnetic powers, and organic adjustments, have all long continued, and probably will still continue to mislead the medical enquirer.

There is affectation in physic as well as in religion. Men will always be found to pride themselves even in appearing to see farther than their fellow mortals. The vulgar things of this sublunary world, and which are seen every day passing around us, will seldom be contemplated by them, or if they are at all considered, it must be in connexion with objects far more sublime, more subtle, and more mysterious. Hence, in the sight of some philosophers, an object becomes often insignificant the moment it becomes comprehensible.

In other parts of the work, we have noticed the doctrine of occult causes more fully. Here we will only repeat what has been observed in other places; that natural causes have ever been the same : statistical ones only vary. On this account, contagious epidemical diseases will prevail much in one country, not in another—in the same country in one age, and not in the succeeding one ; that a strict connexion exists between contagious diseases and the institutions, religious, moral, and political of a people. On the other hand, that no connexion whatever has ever been traced between them and the aspect of the stars, the course of the planets, or the mineralogical, or meteorological arrangements of the earth or heavens; and finally, that it is unphilosophical to admit the operation of hidden causes, not only without proof, but in defiance of reason or analogy.

The diseases of a people are sometimes as transferable as their merchandize, their manners or customs. If a disease be contagious, it will be conveyed from one country to another with as much facility as the manufactures, providing the climate and condition of the people are similar in both. If a disease be not contagious, its conveyance from country to country will just take as long time as the change of manners and customs require.

The mode of conveyance has been mistaken. Dr. Adams, who believes in the Egyptian origin of plague, thus represents it. After observing that the plague of 1348 was more dreadful in England than the one in 1665, and ascribing both to an infectious atmosphere, he adds, " nor is there any reason to doubt that this pestilential atmosphere pervaded *the whole of the East from China.*" In this instance Dr. Adams has mistaken the nature of contagion, which in every case is incapable of extending its power of propagation beyond a few feet or yards from its source. " The baleful influence," says Dr. Currie, " derived to the atmosphere from taking its constant course over extensive swamps of many thousand acres of putrefying vegetable and animal matter has been loosely applied to the same air passing over a human body for a thousandth part of the time and a millionth part of the surface." *(Letter to Dr. Clerk, Clerk's Collection of Papers, &c.)* Yet marsh effluvia themselves could have no such effect on the atmosphere in general, so as to explain the fact here alluded to by Dr. Adams. It admits of a much easier explanation ; for at a time when every science was involved in the obscurity of the darker ages, before Europe was civilized, quarantine adopted, medicine known, and before Gama's brilliant discovery of the passage to India by the

Cape of Good Hope, is it not more reasonable to conclude, that the matter of contagion, like a great deal of our merchandise, was imported from the East, and its effects fiist felt in the principal commercial towns in the West. From Cairo, Bagdad, Aleppo, Smyrna, and Constantinople, it was often conveyed to places that were situated directly in that line of merchandise; as Malta, Venice, Leghorn, Naples, Marseilles, Paris, London, Amsterdam, Vienna, Moscow, &c. &c.

This seems to be the only reasonable explanation that can be given of this, perhaps the most important, fact in the whole history of contagion.

The quotation from Dr. Adams's work is important in another point of view. It serves to shew what influence the doctrine of atmospherics held over enlightened minds, even to a late period, and how well it is adapted to blind us to what is passing around us.

Dr. Adams, before he published his justly celebrated works on epidemics and morbid poisons, must have been well aware of the dreadful ravages the plague had formerly made in Europe; he must have seen the errors committed by the writers who had given accounts of different epidemics, in ascribing their occurrence to atmospheric constitutions, planetary influence, and other natural causes : he must have observed that, in proportion as the evident causes of disease had been removed by civilization advancing, by the adoption of quarantine, and by changing the rout of merchandise from a direct land line to a circuitous water-carriage, the plague disappeared in Europe. Yet all this was not sufficient to disturb his more sublime contemplations.

If it be allowed that the matter of contagion is subject to the same laws which regulate other matters in a similar form, the mode in which the sensible qualities of the atmosphere act upon it seems to admit of explanation.

Moisture in the air may act, not only by influencing the solubility of contagion, as already stated, but, if accompanied with other bodies, by increasing the weight of the atmosphere

c

itself; it must thus be rendered better fitted to suspend other foreign matters.

A pure dry air, as it possesses a less specific gravity than one which is impure and humid, will of course be less able to float a substance perhaps not many degrees lighter than itself; or the air in a very great degree of rarefaction may be unfitted to contain the subtle fluid in a sufficient concentrated form.

"It is well known," says Paris, "that volatile bodies are sooner converted into a gaseous form by the presence of water in the atmosphere. This is strikingly exemplified by the greater rapidity with which limestone is burnt and reduced to quicklime in moist weather, and by the assistance which is rendered in a dry season by placing a pan of water in the ash-pit. So, again, the perfume of flowers is most sensible when the air is humid, as during the fall of the evening dew: for the same reason the stench of putrid ditches and common-sewers is conveyed to the organ of smell much more speedily in Summer previous to rain, when the air is charged with moisture." (See *Pharmacologia*, p. 139.)

Rain will have a different effect from moisture. If rain be heavy and long-continued, the ordinary effects of moisture on volatile bodies here described will be no longer perceptible. Hence the perfumes of flowers and the odours arising from other substances will cease; or, in other words, the atmosphere will be freed from the presence of foreign bodies. The matter of contagion must be subject to the same law. Heavy rains will dilute it or wash it away.

A hard frost will fix the subtle fluid to surrounding objects in the way it does vapours of other kinds. If frost be severe and of long continuance the poison may be altogether destroyed. If, on the other hand, the frost be less severe or shorter in duration, it is probable that the poison, after being sometime suspended in its operation, may be set loose by a thaw, and again become active. A free circulation of air in a place prevents the accumulation of contagion by preventing concentration and carrying it away; while a stagnant state of it is favorable to contagion, in the same way it is known to be to marsh effluvia, simple moisture, or other atmospheric impregnations. High temperature, generally speaking, diminishes the influence of contagion by rarefying the air.

Such seems to be the explanation of the influence of the atmosphere on the agent itself, and, so far as we have here entered into it, our doctrine is supported by facts as well as reason and analogy. We are well aware it will be deemed speculative by some; yet those who act fairly cannot refuse to contagion the same powers and privileges granted by all to other matters which exist in a similar form.

As perfumes or odours can only sensibly affect the atmosphere to a short distance from their source, so the influence of contagion is as certainly confined to a narrower sphere.

The extent to which the atmosphere will be impregnated must depend upon the size and vigour of the impregnating power. A dung-hill will impregnate to a greater extent than a single rose ; many thousands of acres of animal and vegetable corruption, in the form of swamp, than a small pond in a gentleman's garden ; a human body less than the two latter, and so on. But in all cases of this kind, the size even of the largest sources of corruption, bears such an insignificant proportion to the immense expanse of general atmosphere, that contamination to a hurtful extent must be merely local, and therefore confined to a narrow sphere. This is so obvious even to the most common observer, that we deem it necessary to apologize for mentioning it. Yet the fact is not known, or at least properly adverted to, by philosophers, as Dr. Adams' stratum of air extending from China to different parts of Europe, and arising from human bodies, sufficiently demonstrates. The contaminating power of effluvia arising from the human body must be different in patients labouring under the same disease. A man who has a thousand pustules in small-pox, all teeming with infectious matter, must be more dangerous to surrounding objects than one who has only ten. The difference of the power of infection must be still greater in different diseases, and a malady usually restricted to a twenty days' course will form a greater quantity of contagion, *cæteris paribus*, than one which is restricted to a shorter period.

Generally speaking, a greater quantity of contagion is generated in a single person labouring under small-pox than in most other contagious distempers. The contagion of small-pox, being doubly armed, has the power of infecting either by contact or through the medium of the air to a short distance. Its matter adheres better to some substances than to others; and it will infect either in the form of a scab, in that of a limpid fluid, or in a gaseous form, as before stated. The persons most liable to this disease are, besides, placed in a very different condition. As they are, in most instances, children carried in the arms of another person, they are generally either wrapt up in a cloak, or huddled up closely in a cradle. They are thus more closely exposed to the infecting power, at an age, too, when they are most susceptible to all external impression. A soldier manœuvering in the ranks of a regiment, some of whom are infected with plague, typhus, or yellow fever, is placed in a much less dangerous situation. What the mortality in small-pox and the like distempers must have been, when the hot regimen, as it was called, was in vogue, (wrapping the patient up in warm blankets and keeping him in close heated apartments,) is not difficult to conjecture, even if there had been no heart-rending history to record the dreadful tale. Yet we found this horrid practice still prevailing in Greece.

The contagions, no more than any other class of bodies, will be regulated precisely by the same laws. Like the class of gaseous bodies, acids, or neutral salts, they possess properties sufficiently similar to distinguish them as a class, yet each has its individual peculiarities. One is more volatile than another; one more active; another mild one is operated upon by heat, another by cold: some are destroyed by the agency of certain conditions of atmosphere, as moisture, dryness, rest, or motion; others are more independent of such influences: some are more readily conveyed from place to place, &c. &c. In this, however, there is less difference to be observed amongst them than what is observable in some other classes of agents.

The healthy secretions or products of the human body likewise differ much in their appearance and properties. We could no more take one of them as a standard for the others than we can take one of the morbid secretions for an example of the rest. Yet all products of the body, healthy as well as morbid, are formed from the same mass of blood.

The products even of dead matters vary much according to the mode in which they are treated. By the mere regulation of heat and moisture we have sugar at one stage of fermentation, wine from another, and acid or vinegar from a third; and all this from the same substances being subjected to different modes of management. Yet what a vast difference obtains between the beer, spirits, or wine of one manufacturer from that of another, even in cases where the exact same materials have been employed, and where *every possible cure* has been taken to manage them in the same way.

This may give us some faint idea of the powers of the animal system to vary its products in health and disease.

Hitherto we have chiefly alluded to the influence of the atmosphere on the agent, contagion, itself. The effects of certain conditions of atmosphere on the subject exposed now fall to be noticed. Cold, heat, moisture, dryness, &c. affect the soil as well as the seed. The non-contagionists do not seem to have considered this part of the subject with due attention: they too frequently notice the effects of atmospheric changes in relation to earthy or marsh effluvia alone, without taking into their accounts the very marked and obvious effects of the same changes of air on human effluvia.

During a cold and moist state of weather people shut

their doors and windows, and confine themselves more to their houses. The filthy crowded habitations of the poor at such times are frequently so circumstanced as to keep the wretched inmates in a state analogous to disease; for, being unable to afford fire to ventilate or warm their apartments, they have recourse to that heat which is derived from the bodies of each other. When the weather is hot or the atmosphere pure and dry, most of their time is spent out of doors, while more care is taken to ventilate their dwellings. The clothing of the people is likewise different. The very weather which induced them to close their houses compelling them to change their clothing at the same time, as from cotton sometimes washed to woollen never changed, a substance of all others the best adapted to accumulate and preserve human effluvia. What must be the condition of the individuals of a poor family who, from the want of fire or blankets, are compelled to sleep for months together in such clothing. He only who has practised much amongst the poor in our large crowded cities, who has witnessed the parent's anxious look over the helpless, half-starved, and sickly offspring, can form any correct notion of their wretchedness and misery. Need we wonder or complain if Providence has decreed that the diseases which arise thus amongst the poor should recoil upon the rich, as a just punishment for their want of charity? The condition of the poor here alluded to is known to aggravate typhus fever more particularly.

Something may be safely laid to the charge of the atmosphere in predisposing the people to contagious diseases.

Its influence on the form and character of diseases specifically contagious must not be left out of view.

The fever which accompanies the acute contagious diseases is much influenced by temperature and other conditions of air. If it be allowed that the quantity of the morbid product, contagion, generated in an individual labouring under disease, depends in a great measure on the vigour and duration of the morbid action, the cause which produces it, we can readily understand the nature of the atmospheric influence here alluded to.

We have a familiar illustration of this in cases of smallpox. If a patient labouring under this disorder be treated in a hot or impure air, his fever will be aggravated; the effect of which is, that he has the confluent and worst kind of pustules. On the other hand, if he be kept in a cooler atmosphere, his fever will be less violent, the pustules fewer and of a better character. Cold affusion, by lessening fever and destroying the morbid action, arrests at the same time the creative process in scarlet fever, &c.

In very hot seasons we have observed this last disease attended with more eruption on the skin; sometimes with extensive vesications or blisters, proving fatal in forty-eight hours from the first appearance of fever. At other times it is scarcely a febrile disease, or as Sydenham observed, " a disease of any kind." On this account, Dr. Adams, in his celebrated work on morbid poisons, recommends, that children who have never had measles or scarlet fever should be exposed to their contagion in mild seasons. Every contagious disease has its favourite season, as we shall afterwards see. But instances are on record of all of them appearing out of their usual time. A proof that the conditions of atmosphere, so much noticed by writers, were accessory, not essential causes. They never, therefore, can stand in the relation of cause and effect.

When contagious diseases do occur out of their usual times, or even otherwise, they sometimes put on forms characteristic of the seasons in which they happen to make their appearance.

In Spring the same disease will partake more of the inflammatory disposition; in Summer or Autumn, it will have a bilious or putrid cast; in Winter, catarrhal, and so on.

It does not seem to require the aid of the occult sciences to account for some of these effects of season on the human body. In Winter, when the cold invigorates the system, sharpens a man's appetite, but diminishes his perspiration, and sometimes his exercise, he will become plethoric.

When the heat is first felt in Spring, and extends the volume of blood without diminishing its quantity, this overfulness of the vascular system will be most perceptible. The sudden changes from hot to cold weather, for which this season is so remarkable, must increase this inflammatory tendency. Hence arises the wish for bleeding in the Spring.

In the course of the Summer the system becomes reduced in different ways, and by evident causes. It is relaxed by heat, fatigued by exercise, and wasted by excessive perspiration. A great proportion of the vegetable kingdom, having arrived at maturity, begins to decay in Autumn. As animal and vegetable decomposition advances, the human system, before debilitated and relaxed by the Summer's heat, will now more readily participate in the general putrid tendency. Autumn does not possess the equable temperature of Summer. In its variableness it resembles Spring, but with this difference, that, in the former, the changes of weather are from a hot to a colder; whereas, in the latter, they are more frequently from a cold to a warmer state of atmosphere. As it is neither steady cold nor uniformly hot weather which proves unfriendly to the animal system (the body adapting itself in time to either), but sudden changes from the one to the other, which do not afford time for this adaptation; so Summer and Winter, in many countries, are more healthy seasons than Spring or Autumn. The latter, for reasons given, is generally the most sickly. Obstructed perspiration, however vulgar the notion may appear to be to some philosophers, is, we are convinced, the chief cause of disease in every climate under the sun. In cold and temperate regions, when the perspiration is suddenly checked by any means, Nature tries to relieve herself by an increased flow of blood to the organs of the chest and throat. Catarrh, croup, sore throat, pneumonia, pleurisy, and phthisis, are therefore the most common diseases of such latitudes.

But who are the principal sufferers from such complaints?—those who are least on their guard to provide against changes of weather; the young, vain, headstrong, and inexperienced. We found the same cause produce very different effects in tropical climates.

Here the usual mode of relief adopted by Nature is, by a determination of blood to the abdominal viscera, as the liver, stomach, and bowels; hence, liver complaints, cholera, bilious attacks, dysentery, and diarrhœa will supervene, while the before-mentioned diseases of the chest will be seldom observed. In a country possessing a climate between these two, or the high temperate, as it is called, the prevailing diseases will neither be of the one kind nor the other, but a mixture of both. In the Mediterranean, therefore, phthisis, and other complaints of the chest are met with in the variable season of the year, while the diseases of tropical climates are not unfrequent during hot weather.

The chest affections, too, for obvious reasons, prevail more in persons arrived from colder climates than in natives. So do all other distempers arising from climate. The determinations of blood to particular organs will be attended with different effects according to climate. In a cold or temperate region, where the fibre is more rigid and the system more vigorous, they will be followed with a correspondent vigour in their action.

In a tropical climate, where the system is relaxed, and somewhat weakened, the action will be chronic. To speak professionally, the one is congestive, the other inflammatory. Hence, the acute diseases of the one, and the chronic affections of the other. It must be undertood we are here speaking only of the effects of climate without reference to the two great causes of disease—marsh and human effluvia. These two produce every where a peculiar train of symptoms, differing, under ordinary circumstances, uniformly from each other; but need we wonder if the diseases arising from both put on some of the characteristics of climate and season?

Need we wonder if both the marsh and contagious disease of a hot climate be frequently attended with yellowness of the skin, disorganization of the liver or stomach, congestions of the head, a tendency to putrefaction in the fluids, &c. ? Need we wonder if the contagious disease of a temperate climate, typhus, be there accompanied with acute inflammations of the chest or brain ? Under ordinary circumstances, the fever attendant on a contagious disease, is always a continued fever, that arising from marsh effluvia, remittent or intermittent; but we have good evidence to prove that a disease, specifically contagious, and alike contagious in every climate in which it prevails, though not in every season, sometimes assumes that form of fever which characterises a marsh disease.

This circumstance, which appears to be purely accidental, has nevertheless a powerful effect on enlightened minds, at the present day; for, if we mistake not, it was a case of typhus fever terminating in an intermittent, which induced Dr. Armstrong to doubt the contagious nature of this disease, and to attribute its origin, in some places, to marshy or earthy exhalations; a doctrine which is now taught in London in some schools.

That typhus does sometimes terminate in an intermittent form of fever, is an undoubted fact, but we have observed it to do so by the mere force of remedies in places where an intermittent fever would be looked upon as a rare curiosity: where, in fact, not the smallest suspicion could possibly have been entertained of marsh or marsh-like exhalations. That typhus and other contagious diseases will be exasperated by such like exhalations we have not any doubt. Accordingly, Sir Gilbert Blane mentions, in his dissertations, that "when typhus poison exists in a slight degree, a warm climate dissipates it; but, when in a concentrated state, it is exasperated by the heat of the atmosphere, *and by palludal (marsh) exhalations.*"

The same distinguished author adds " if the sphere of infection extended to the whole atmosphere, there could be no more danger in the closest approach than at the greatest distance." P. 221.

Plague is also influenced by marsh effluvia. According to Sir James M'Grigor, " when the plague first broke out in the Indian army on the expedition to Egypt, the crowded hospitals of the 61st and 88th regiments were, from the first, attacked with typhous symptoms ; while those from the Bengal Volunteer Battalion, and the other corps *near the marshes of El Hamed, evinced uniformly an intermittent or remittent type*; and those that occurred during the cold and rainy months of December and January, an inflammatory character ; after which, as the weather became warmer, the disease, at Cairo, Ghiza, Boulac, and the Isthmus of Suez, wore the form of a mild continued fever."—*See Medical Statistics.*

Many writers mention similar facts regarding plague. It is a disease so liable to be disguised by the influence of season and other causes, that there is scarcely an instance of an epidemic plague on record, being recognised by medical men at its first breaking out. The exact same thing has taken place in numerous cases of epidemic yellow fever. Yet it was in their external forms only they differed ; for all their essential peculiarities existed in each from the beginning. To use the words of Sir Thomas Maitland, " the plague was the plague, the whole plague, and nothing but the plague."— *See his excellent Letter to Earl Bathurst, on the Plague of Malta, Corfu, &c.*

Some are disposed to deny that a true contagious fever can ever be influenced or altered in its form by marsh effluvia ; alleging, as a reason for scepticism, that two diseased actions are *always* incompatible with each other, and therefore cannot take place in the same person at the same time. The matter seems to stand thus :—The human system is susceptible of a vast variety of external impressions. As some of those are friendly to health, and others unfavourable, so some of them excite a morbid action in the system, which assists or aggravates other morbid actions of a similar kind, while others oppose or are wholly incompatible. On what other principle can we explain the phenomena of health and disease? On what other principle can the marked effects of remedies employed in the cure be explained?

We cure one disease by exciting another in the system, by means of the remedies we employ. If the action of the medicine happens to be incompatible with the morbid action it will succeed in the cure. If the operation of the medicine excites a similar action it may aggravate the very disorder we intended to cure, and it may even add another train of symptoms in some degree foreign to its ordinary characteristics. So does the matter stand with diseases themselves. Pregnancy arrests the progress of consumption of the lungs, also of sivvens;* it increases the tendency to mania, indigestion, hysteria, &c. Scrofula aggravates the symptoms of syphilis and renders it difficult of cure; a scorbutic taint, those of itch; and we have observed scurvy, dysentery and liver complaint in the same individual at the same time, each tending to aggravate the other. A fever arising from cold, insolation, or marsh miasmata, will become contagious under certain circumstances being added to aggravate its nature. By the like means, an intermittent fever will become continued at one time, and remittent at another, according as causes are added or taken away, or as they happen to be compatible or incompatible with each other.

It is true, two acute contagious diseases will not affect the general system at the same time. There is however, a very great difference between the nature of the diseased action produced by contagion and marsh effluvia. Contagion once applied, accumulates in the system by means of the very action it excites. To suppose then, that two different contagions could operate simultaneously in the same body, is to

---

* See Adams on Morbid Poisons.

suppose that the same organ or set of organs are capable of performing two distinct functions at the same time. As well might we expect the liver to secrete bile and urine or semen with the same means, or with the same organization. The action produced by marsh effluvia does not accumulate the cause in the system on which it operates. It is an expulsive process merely that takes place; not a creative and expulsive, as in the case of contagion. The cause, marsh poison, therefore, may be supposed to be diminished in the system by the very action it excites. As it is derived from without the body, not generated within it, the fever it excites must also vary in its force according to the force or degree of concentration of the poison.

This is also the case in contagion; but a cause which exists in the system itself, and which is there accumulated by its own power, must be attended with a fever more uniform and continued than a cause derived from without, and depending on a number of adventitious circumstances, over which the body has no control. The febrile disease arising from contagion is in every instance restricted to a short course, and the action in general cannot be repeated by the same kind of poison.

The febrile disease caused by marsh effluvia is in no instance restricted in the length of its course; but as both the duration of each paroxysm, and the form or type of the disease itself depend on the variable cause from without, the fever may continue for an indefinite time, and be repeated in the same person, or it may be altered, or modified as often as the cause is applied or altered, or modified in its power.

This explains the reason why, in cases where both marsh and human effluvia conspire in exciting febrile action in the same person at the same time, the fever from contagion ceases (being more restricted in duration) while the marsh fever continues.

Again, if marsh poison and the poison of contagion unite in exciting in the system an expulsive process by similar fevers, we can have no difficulty in understanding why that

system, which has both causes to expel at one and the same
time, having a greater task to perform, must be more burdened
in its operation of relief than if one of the agents.had been
in operation. We have thus endeavoured to explain some of
the modifications produced by atmospheric influence and
marsh poison on disease. Whether these explanations be
satisfactory or not, the facts remain the same.

That different diseases of a season, whether contagious or
not, will often assume something of the same character when
any remarkable .quality of the atmosphere is in excess, is an
observation which has been made by authors from the earliest
periods, at which those diseases were known.

The disease which happens to be most favoured by season,
and other circumstances, will prevail most for a time. In
other words, it will be the *epidemic* of the season. The others
being less favoured will often decline as it gains ground, and
thus leave the field to the conqueror. In seasons, where no
one is able to take up the whole field to himself, several
diseases may appear in the same season, and it will be observed, that one of them has the ascendancy. In this case,
the minor diseases of the season will wear something of the
garb or uniform and follow some of the motions of the com-
manding officer or chief epidemic of the year.

Thucydides, as early as the plague of Athens, observes,
" Enimvèro, annus ille ut confessione fere omnium constat,
maxime immunis fuit aliorum morborum, quod si quisquis
alio prius laborabet, is morbus in hunc convertabatur."

In the age of our illustrious Sydenham, the contagious
diseases in Britain, seem to have maintained a perpetual
struggle for supremacy. Sometimes small-pox was feugle-
man, sometimes plague ; at others, both these tyrants left
the field to a third of an inferior rank, which, after reigning
some time with a despotic sway, was again superseded by a
fourth.*

* According to Sydenham, fevers then constituted two thirds of mortal

" Morbi præsentes," says Hippocrates, " a præterita tem-
porum conditione fluunt; accipiunt vero etiam differentiam
a conditione præsentis, quare utriusque oportet habere ra-
tionem."

It must be here remarked, that Hippocrates restricted his
ideas to atmospheric constitutions alone; but as he could not
account for the prevalence of particular diseases of one year,
by referring it to the sensible qualities of the air of that
year, he was led to ascribe it to the previous year's constitution.

Sydenham has evidently followed in his footsteps—so have
many authors since their time. It was this inability to explain epidemic diseases on the principles of the sensible
qualities of the air alone, which has given rise to so much
error. Dr. Jackson, one of the most distinguished noncontagionists in yellow fever, observes, " epidemic influence, as
already observed, is fundamentally different from the common
influence connected with the revolutions of the seasons."
It is at the same time true, that it (yellow fever) very often
assumes the features of morbid action which belongs to the
season of the year in which it happens to occur. The fact
is an important one, and in illustration of it, I take the opportunity to state, that the forms of diseased action were
different at different periods during the whole continuance
of the epidemic which prevailed in Brimstone Hill in the
year 1812. In the months of March and April, when the
weather was dry, *the cold considerable* during the night, *the
heat great* during the day, the morbid action was generally
such as is termed *inflammatory,* sometimes suppurative,
sometimes in such excess as to be gangrenous—the stomach
and head the principal organs affected : in May and June,
when the weather was *mild* with moderate showers of rain,
the symptoms *were less violent* in appearance, the mode of

diseases, and eight out of every nine that died, were cut off by febrile
diseases.

action sometimes characterised by adhesion between contiguous parts, and effusion of watery fluids into cavities—the
head and stomach the organs which principally suffered."—
Jackson on Febrile Diseases, p. 22.

We see then, yellow fever, influenced by season, as well
as all other contagious diseases. How Dr. Jackson thought
this fact more important in yellow fever may be surmised
from his wish to ascribe it to season alone, not to contagion.
He accordingly points out its dependance on weather, as if it
had been something peculiar to this disease, instead of being
common in small-pox, measles, scarlet fever, plague, typhus,
&c.

But as Dr. Jackson, no more than Hippocrates, Sydenham,
or indeed any one else, was able to explain the whole phenomena by season alone; so, like them, he was forced to add a
hidden influence. Need it be repeated, that no natural cause
connected directly or indirectly with the atmosphere, is of
itself sufficient to account for the history of contagious diseases.

Plague, small-pox, scarlet fever, typhus, and venereal disease, have been chief epidemics in Britain, within the period
of well-authenticated history. Plague and small-pox have
both been beaten off the field: syphilis seems fast going,
while typhus and scarlet fever can scarcely be recognized as
the same diseases. Does it require a knowledge of atmospherics to tell why plague has disappeared; why small-pox
became first modified in its virulence by a change from the
hot to the cool regimen; why it was still further changed in
its character by inoculation, and became a rare and insignificant malady by vaccination? Does it require any such aid
to explain why the petechial typhus of the older authors, and
the low nervous fever of Cullen, which he characterized by
the distinguishing sign " calor parum auctus," have now
given way to one attended with more heat of skin and with
inflammatory symptoms, requiring bleeding. In the same
way scarlet fever, which was scarcely accounted a disease in

the age of Sydenham, is now also one of greater excitement and danger. Does it require any knowledge of the atmosphere, or of what we call topographical causes, to tell why the venereal disease, which was at first attended with fever, became chronic, and is at length so much changed in its appearance as scarcely to be recognized as the same disease? We think decidedly not; let us hope, then, that the noseless age of syphilis is now passed, and that a person without the promontory of the face from this cause, will in future be as rarely seen as one pitted with small-pox.

The Rise, Progress, and Decline of Epidemics further Explained.

We shall next make an attempt to apply the principles laid down to the epidemic plague which raged in West Barbary, in 1799, an excellent account of which has been given by James Gray Jackson, Esq. then British Consul at Mogodore.

This is to be preferred to any history given by a medical man, as it cannot be supposed that the author was misled by any favourite theory. The disease was, besides, uninfluenced by insusceptibility of persons arising from previous attacks of the same malady, no plague having been in West Barbary for a great length of time.

It has been remarked by many writers, that *when plague attacks a large city, a greater proportion of the persons seized at the beginning die, but that the number infected is small.* These facts may be thus explained. A greater proportion of the persons seized die, because those only who are most susceptible are at first attacked. Accordingly, Mr. Jackson remarks, that " young, healthy, and robust persons of full stamina, were for the most part attacked first, then women and children, and lastly, thin, sickly, emaciated and old persons." Young, healthy, and robust persons of a full stamina were the most likely to suffer from the following

reasons :—1st, From leading an active life and bustling about
in every direction, they were most exposed to the causes of
disease.   2nd, From their constitutions being then free
from other diseases, they were most liable when exposed.
3d, Their systems were capable, when once infected, of going
into a more violent morbid action.   Whence the greater proportion of deaths at the beginning.

The small number of persons infected, might depend on
the following circumstances. 1st, The contagion is small
in quantity; of course not generally diffused. 2nd, A number
of persons are not susceptible from having their systems
pre-occupied with other diseases. 3d, The season most
favourable to the disease has not arrived.

" In Old Fez," adds Mr. J. " it broke out in the month of
April, and soon communicated itself to the new city ; carrying
off one or two the first day ; three or four the second day ;
six or eight the third ; increasing progressively, till the mortality amounted to two in the hundred of the aggregate
population ; continuing with unabated violence ten, fifteen,
or twenty days; being of longer duration in *old* than in
new towns; then diminishing in a progressive proportion
from *one thousand* a day to nine hundred, then to eight
hundred, and so on till it disappeared."   Whilst it raged
in the town of Mogodore, a small village (Diabet) situated
about two miles south-east of that place *remained uninfected, although the communication was open between them ;*
on *the thirty-fourth* day, however, after its first appearance at Mogodore, this village was discovered to be infected, and the disorder raged with great violence, making
dreadful havoc among the human species for *twenty-one
days,* carrying off during that period *one hundred* persons
out of *one hundred and thirty-three,* the original population
of the village before the plague visited it; none died after
this, and those who were infected recovered in the course of
a month or two.

All the villages dispersed through the extensive Shelluh

province of Haha shared a similar or a worse fate. In one village, consisting of a population of six hundred persons, *only four escaped.* Other villages which had contained four or five hundred, had only seven or eight survivors.

The population of the cities are thus given :—Morocco, 270,000 ; Mogodore, 10,000 ; Fez, Old and New, 380,000 ; Teroodant, 25,000. When the disease was at its height, Morocco lost 1,000 persons each day; Teroodant lost 800 a day; and the populous cities of Old and New Fez diminished their population 12 or 1500 each day. There died during the above periods, in Morocco, 50,000; in Fez, 65,000 ; in Mogodore; 4,509, and in Saffy, 5,000 ; in all 124,500.

In these extensive cities the mortality was so great, that, the living not having time to bury the dead, the bodies were deposited or thrown altogether into large holes, which, when nearly full, were covered over with earth.

The other circumstances connected with the rise, progress, and decline of this famous epidemic, admit of explanation, although it was never ascertained from whence it had been introduced. The climate is described as being extremely healthy, so that the plague had not been known in the memory of any one then alive.

1st. *It therefore appeared amongst a people whose constitutions were unprotected by any previous attack.*

Mr. Jackson thought this disease somewhat different in its nature from the Turkish plague ; yet he describes in his cases the same leading characteristics, viz. buboes, carbuncles, black spots on the skin, like grains of gunpowder, &c. His ground for believing them different, was merely that the Barbary plague *was more active* than the one of Constantinople ; a circumstance at once accounted for by the more frequent occurrence of plague in the latter city, thus destroying the susceptibility of its inhabitants.

By Mr. Jackson's account, it appears that even the Arabs were aware that it could not be again epidemic in Barbary, for a length of time, though their reasons for thinking so are not stated. " *Agreeably to this opinion it did not re-appear the second year.*"

2nd. The crowded cities and narrow streets of even the villages in Barbary, were well calculated to spread a contagious disease, though only communicable by contact.

" The streets of Mogodore," Mr. J. says " are narrow, the houses having few windows towards the streets. Horses, camels, and other beasts, live together with men, women, and children indiscriminately, in the southern provinces. In Morocco, the streets are nearly filled with ruined houses, which have gone to decay. In the Jews' quarter heaps of dung and other filth are seen as high as the houses. Every body is anxious how to conceal his wealth, hence the houses are concealed by a wall." The villages in Barbary are much like the cities in these respects. What, then, but an extremely healthy climate, and a dry sandy soil, could possibly preserve them from destruction.

3d. The total ignorance of the people as to the cause of plague, would have prevented them taking any precautions against its violence, had their religion permitted them to use means.

4th. " There prevails along the coast of West Barbary," says Mr. J, " a trade-wind, which begins to blow in the months of May, June, July, and August, with little intermission. It was apprehended that the influence of this trade-wind, added to the superstitious opinion of the plague ceasing on St. John's day, would stop, or at least sensibly diminish the mortality, but no such thing happened ; the wind did set in as it invariably does at St. John's day ; the disorder, however, increased rather than diminished at that period."

No such changes of weather will effectually arrest a contagious disease like plague, *where every other circumstance favours its propagation.*

5th. Mr. Jackson continues—" Some persons were of opinion that the decrease of mortality did not originate from a decrease in the miasma, but from a decrease of subjects to prey upon.

" This is a plausible idea, but admitting it to be just, how are we to explain the almost invariable fatality of the disorder when at its height, and the comparative innocence of it when on the decline ; for then the chance to those who had it was, that they would recover, and survive the malady."

This is accounted for by many circumstances afterwards to be noticed. Here, however, it may be observed, that Mr. J. has himself partly explained it. " The thin, sickly, emaciated and old persons," were not only the least susceptible, but their constitutions, when attacked, were incapable of entering into that strong morbid action which was observed in the persons first seized, viz. " young, healthy, robust persons of full stamina."

When the contagion became extended, and in fact nearly universally diffused, the disease disappeared.

This can be explained on the principle, that all those who were liable to its influence had already gone through the disease. In proportion to the activity of the contagion must be the duration of the epidemic.

Where a thousand houses are crowded together, a conflagration will run more rapidly through them than if they had been placed at a greater distance from each other. If, after it has gone through them and ceased, fresh fuel be brought to the place, the flame will be again renewed.

This was observed in the present instance, for according to Mr. Jackson, " families that had gone to the country to avoid the infection, on returning home, *when all infection had apparently ceased, were generally attacked and died.*" So we see that the contagion, which had no power over 220,000 persons still alive in Morocco, 5,500 in Mogodore, 315,000, in Old and New Fez, and a large number in Teroodant and Saffy, had yet the power of destroying susceptible persons when brought within its reach. A singular instance of this happened at Mogodore, " where," (says Mr. J.) " *after the mortality had subsided*, a corps of troops arrived from Teroodant, where the plague had been raging, but had likewise subsided. These troops, after remaining three days at Mogodore, (the usual time for infection manifesting itself in the human body), were attacked with the disease, and it raged extensively amongst them *for about a month*, while it carried off about *two-thirds* of their original number." Here then, we have an instance of a corps of troops, which had either been not exposed to contagion in the town they left, or were not susceptible to its influence, which, nevertheless, became instantly liable on removal to another town, where the mortality had ceased, leaving 5,500 persons still alive. Had the whole remaining inhabitants and soldiers removed from Mogodore at the month's end, when plague ceased amongst all, and been replaced by an equal number of strangers, who had never before suffered from its influence, the epidemic, we are convinced, would have again rekindled and continued in force until that season had arrived known to be unfavourable to its influence, *viz.*, hard frost, heavy rains, &c.

Strangers, as it has long been remarked by authors, are peculiarly liable to epidemic, plague, yellow fever, &c.

When the strangers happen to be natives of a different climate, just or lately arrived in the place where it is begun, they not only labour under that state of excitement which the climate occasions, but they are exposed at the very same time to a new and powerful influence; in other words, they are exposed to two agents at the same time, neither of which existed in their own country. Hence, if a thousand children, natives of the South Sea Islands, were brought to a town in Britain, small-pox, measles, scarlet fever, or hooping-cough, might be epidemic amongst them, at a time when those diseases were scarcely believed to exist amongst the inhabitants themselves. Natives of a cool or temperate climate, arriving suddenly in one which is hot, stand in a much worse situation than persons attacked with a disease in Spring or Autumn, in their own climate. Yet, we have shewn, that Spring and Autumn are the most unhealthy seasons.

Again, who are strangers ? They are persons who have been induced to travel from motives of curiosity or interest, very frequently from both. In what way is curiosity satisfied, information obtained, or interest promoted ? The answer is just as easy, by communication and intercourse. Strangers are persons, too, having no settled place of abode. On this account they live in lodging-houses, where they meet other strangers similarly situated as themselves ; a sailor meeting a sailor, a merchant a merchant, and so on. In such houses, they often sit at the same table, occupy the same sofa or chair, sup with a spoon, or eat with a knife and fork, before used by another; wipe their hands with the same cloth, drink out of the jug; hand round the same snuff-box, and some-times, (for they are not all persons of fortune, delicacy, or fashion,) sleep in the same room, very often in the same bed: all this with people they never saw before, nor may never see after.

Need we wonder, then, if those quarters of a large city where lodging-houses most abound, are remarkable as being those first infected? Lodging-houses of this description are generally situated in the low dirty narrow streets of large commercial sea-port towns ; in other words, in places most convenient for the shipping. Yet, this last circumstance has been laid hold on by the non-contagionists, and adduced as a proof of marsh effluvia.

Strangers, having once sallied from their dangerous abodes, may be seen in every quarter of a large town, in the course of a few hours. The man of curiosity impatiently walks to the most public places. He visits the churches, banks, courts of law, museums and markets, during the day; plays, balls, routs, masquerades, in the evening; at all which places, he comes in close contact with a hundred persons just as curious as himself. The very man who describes to him or his party, the pictures in a gallery of paintings, or the monuments in a church or church-yard, is, in half an hour afterwards, repeating his well-known harangue to another party of amateurs. The merchant, though somewhat differently employed, comes in contact with as many persons in as short a time. Sometimes he is selling, sometimes buying; but, when he first lands with his cargo, he is generally a seller. From the Custom-house he goes to the Exchange, banks, markets, and shops, and his goods, soon spreading in every direction, are replaced by other wares. The sailor, though less prompted by curiosity, interest, or a desire for information, is by no means the least dangerous animal of the three. In a short time, he is in every quarter of the town; he looks at every thing, and does every thing, without being able to tell the reason why; nor can he tell next day where he has been, who he spoke with, or what he saw.

The first appearance of epidemic plagues and yellow fever, has been frequently dated from the arrival of a fleet in a port. As fleets and ships have been blamed for importing those diseases, in many cases where the crews or crew had been healthy till their arrival, the non-contagionists adduce this fact as a proof that such diseases arise from the mere effects of climate on unseasoned constitutions. Had such epidemics been always confined to the new comers, the evidence in favour of this opinion would have been strong. People suddenly exposed to the influence of climate and unhealthy locality at the same time, run as great risk as those who are brought under the influence of climate and contagion. The result, however, would be different in the two cases. In both, the disease would appear first, and rage to a greater extent amongst strangers, as has been already explained. In both cases, the arrival of a fleet would increase the danger to natives of the place, as well as to the strangers themselves. The places of public amusement are thrown open on the arrival of a fleet, and private visiting is increased to a wonderful degree. Races, routes, balls, masquerades, plays and private parties are given on shore,* some of which are returned on ship-board. Hence the question of the lady at St. Helena, who seriously asked a British officer, " if London was not dull when the China fleet left it." Similar changes take place in the ships. The sailors, on their arrival in port, are at once exposed to greater fatigue, in unloading or loading during the day. Many articles of merchandize and clothing are called into requisition for the first time, during the men's service on board; the sailors of one ship visit those of others also for the first time, both on shore and in their ships, &c.

The natural consequence of all this is sufficiently evident; the bad effects of irregular living, late hours, crowded assemblies, exposure to the sun by day and the dews by night, cannot be mistaken in either case. So far then the evidence in favour of climate, season, and unhealthy locality is as strong, if not stronger, than that in favour of contagion.

If in any case, however, the disease be recognized as a stranger, as well as the sailors, amongst whom it first appeared; and, if in addition to this, the ship or ships to which they belong, have just arrived from a country where the disease is known to prevail more than it does in any other climate, then every one who can distinguish right from wrong, truth from falsehood, or reason from folly, must allow that the evidence is in favour of importation. Any of the following circumstances will strengthen this evidence.

We happened to be present at the splendid fancy ball given by Colonel Fitzclarence and the officers of the 7th Fusileers, at Malta, in April, 1829. Upwards of 400 persons sat down to supper. The costume of the reign of Queen Elizabeth seemed to be the order of the night; but, from Obadiah Prim, to young ladies who looked prim enough, there was almost every variety of character present. The iron-cased champion, the brawny Albanian, the turbaned Turk, the Tartaned warrior, the camp strippling, and accoutred dragoon, mixed with princes and pensioners, counts and cardinals, quakers and quack-doctors, lawyers and limbs of the law, indiscriminately. In short, the entertainment was of the first order, mental, alimental, and complimental. If plague had existed, however, it must have been likewise instrumental in spreading the seeds of disease.

1st. The existence, though not in an epidemic form, of the same disease in the place from which the ship came, during her stay there, or before her departure.

2d. The appearance of the disease on board her, soon after arriving at the sickly port, and at a time when the crew were healthy.

3d. Its continuance on board during the passage from one place to the other.

4th. The first persons seized belonging to the port at which she has arrived, being those who had had the first communication with the sickly ship. The above circumstances all conspiring, would make the proof of importation complete, excepting some other evident cause of the disease is discovered on board.

5th. The relations and visitants of the first persons taken ill being soon after attacked with the same disease, although they had never been on board, or near the suspected ship.

6th. The slow and gradual progress of the disease on shore, multiplying from two to four, from four to eight, from eight to sixteen, till a considerable proportion of the inhabitants of the port had gone through the disease.

7th. A great mortality amongst natives of the place, as well as amongst strangers, though not in the same proportion.

8th. Its attacking persons indiscriminately, except with regard to communication with the sick, or things before in contact; *viz.*, the temperate and intemperate, the regular liver as well as those who had engaged in the riot and dissipation before described; even though it should attack the latter in a greater proportion, or more violent degree.

9th. The increase of the disease, when intercourse with the sick is increased, or connexion with things before in contact with them, and its decrease when such intercourse or connexion is decreased. We consider this of itself complete proof of the contagious nature of any disease, even although it should not take place at all times, or under every circumstance alike.

The greater prevalence of epidemic diseases amongst strangers, is not the only circumstance the non-contagionists have pressed into their service. Epidemics have been sometimes observed to break out amongst relations, living in different quarters of the town, at, or near the same time. Those who have witnessed the conduct of strangers, on their first arrival in a place, will not be surprised at this, even if the persons so taken ill had not been related. The aerial theorists, however, explain it on the principle of similarity of constitutions observed or supposed to exist amongst persons nearly related by blood to each other; they leave out altogether the greater probability of intercourse between such relations. We shall suppose a thing by no means unlikely, that one of the strangers, prompted by the ties of relationship, friendship, or from interest, called, on his arrival in port, at the house of an individual; he is almost certain, in either of these cases, to be carried straight to the houses of some of the relations of the individual on whom he called. May not a person convey contagion to others, though in perfect health at the time himself? May not the goods he sells or exchanges, or the presents he gives away, do the same thing? Intercourse in a large town, does not always depend on proximity. Very frequently, next neighbours do not exchange visits for years; sometimes they do not know each other's names or occupations. Occasionally, epidemic diseases are irregular and whimsical in their mode of procedure; they often spread for a time in one direction chiefly, then suddenly change their course to another. At one time they travel with the wind, but in an opposite direction soon after. They frequently prefer one side of a street, or a particular quarter of a town. Sometimes they do not appear in the town for a time, but make nearly a circle round it. Having performed this office in the suburbs or outskirts, they suddenly take a turn to the country by a favourite rout, then return directly to the centre of the town, which is now infected for the first time during the rage of that epidemic. In what way can this be explained, but by referring to that whimsical and capricious being, man, himself.

Smugglers, thieves, vagabonds, and vagrants of all descriptions, have been carriers and importers of contagion in every country. Few of those persons are regulated by law or rule of any kind. Beggars are said to travel with the wind generally; pedlars will not be fond of travelling against it; gypsies have never been remarkable for the regularity of their procedure. As smugglers, thieves, and vagrants have reasons for keeping out of the view of the police, many of them being banished from the towns, they take up their abodes in the suburbs or outskirts, where they are beyond the bounds of police, and where the want of lamps is favourable to their views. Suburbs are chiefly inhabited by two very opposite classes of people; persons from the country, and persons from the town. The former are attracted to towns to spend their money, educate their children, or put them to trades and professions. They often prefer the suburbs on account of the air being purer, house rents cheaper, exemption from town burdens, and being, as they express it, both in town and country. Besides, they believe their children run a less risk of temptation from vice or bad example. A considerable proportion of those from town, on the other hand, are persons, who, as the phrase is, have outrun the constable in different shapes; too well known in every quarter of the town, they remove to obscure parts of the suburbs, amongst strangers to whom they are not known. Many of these persons prowl about the outskirts in every direction during the night, where, favoured by the darkness, and absence of police, they commit all kinds of depredations.

Suppose, then, a criminal, just liberated from jail, where his clothes have become impregnated with the seeds of disease, is banished the city, and goes to haunt with his numerous friends in the suburbs, who could answer for the regularity of his actions, or tell what rout he will take ? Again, a beggar-woman, who lives in the suburbs, borrows a child ill of small-pox, for the purpose of exciting charity; she cannot beg in town, but proceeds in a circular course round it; and, after going this round, she travels directly to the first village in the country. The disease, in this case, would observe the tract of the woman; first round the town, then to the village in the country by the same rout, and, once spread in the village, it would be readily brought back to town by the villagers, who, not being like the beggar proscribed the bounds of police, would carry it to its centre.

The greater partiality of epidemic diseases to one side of a street depends upon difference of intercourse and communication. In most great commercial towns a marked difference may be observed between one side of a principal street and another. Such is the difference in this respect, that, in innumerable instances, the shops of one side let for double the rent of those of the other, even although the accommodation should be similar.

Such is our plain explanation of the occasional whimsical procedure of epidemical diseases. Those who imagine that a contagious disease should, like a volcano, vomit out its flame in all points of the compass alike, might as well compare a common conflagration to a volcano, and expect that the small spark of fire which kindles one should spread in all directions alike, without reference to the fuel which supplies it. A contagion, like small-pox, often spreads rapidly in the villages in Britain. The inhabitants are not so much crowded together as the people in large towns, and the circulation of air is freer; but these advantages are more than counterbalanced by the habit of family visiting being more general. Every individual in a village is known to every other individual. No sooner is a person taken ill of a dangerous disease, than the news becomes known from one end to the other, and all the friends and gossips of the place pay their visits of ceremony or condolence.

If a contagion happens to be less portable or more volatile, it will not spread in villages so much as in towns, particu-

larly in a 'hot climate. Where, however, the houses of villages are as much crowded together as those in the towns,
as is the case in Barbary, then the disease will spread rapidly.
Diseases arising from malaria will likewise be observed sometimes to prevail more on one side of a street—a circumstance
as easily explained as that the one side should have the sun
in the morning, the other in the afternoon. The stone of the
houses built on one side, though of the same age and same
material, nay, even built by the same individual, has a different colour from difference of exposure. In like manner,
the north side of a tree can always be known on inspection.
We know, however, of no possible way by which a disease
arising from an aerial cause alone can be increased, when intercourse with those sick of it is increased, and diminished
when such intercourse is diminished; excepting in cases
where such intercourse caused greater fatigue or anxiety.

Events of great importance to mankind frequently arise
from the most trivial and ordinary causes. Thus, a beggar's
blanket may depopulate a city, the mistress of the world; or,
by cutting short a single life, may even affect the destiny of
a whole nation. Cromwell fell a victim to marsh miasmata.
The health of Napoleon was affected for years, by having
seized the ramrod of a piece of artillery at the seige of Toulon,
at which he had seen an artilleryman killed in the act of
ramming home. Yet few great events happen without efforts
being made to connect them with something deemed more
worthy of themselves; the spirit of prophecy and weather-
wisdom is instantly awakened, and the most ordinary circumstances are sure to be noted down and exaggerated to account
for them. The following have been recorded by authors on
epidemic diseases, and brought in as proof of the existence
of some unusual and mysterious agency.

Domestic animals, such as cows, horses, cats, dogs, birds
in cages, in short, part of all under confinement within doors,
have sometimes been observed to sicken or die during the
rage of an epidemic; women with child miscarried; iron,

steel, and other polished metals corroded; leather become mouldy; clothes mothed and spoiled; beef, &c. putrefied; cheese mited; butter turned rancid; milk soured; the sky had a blood-red cast; the horizon an iron-bound appearance; the sun set every night in an unusual way; the very earth cracked or yawned, as if for its prey; the grass was alive with grasshoppers; the air was darkened with clouds of flies, and other insects; frogs croaked in the ponds, and sparrows, robins, and other small birds disappeared from the place. Such is a specimen of the frightful catalogue in the chapter of accidents, more or less of which have been noted down particularly by the older writers on epidemics. They have likewise been brought forward by some of the moderns of great learning and distinguished rank, in proof of what is called, for the want of a more definable name, epidemic influence : that is, something not referable to the sensible qualities of the atmosphere, or to the effects of season. That these appearances have generally been exaggerated through fear, ignorance, and superstition, can scarcely be doubted, when we remember at how late a period the laws against sorcery and witchcraft were put in force in England.* Sir Gilbert Blane found an instance on record, in the Tower of London, where a man was tried and executed for burning coals, it having been deemed, in older times, injurious to the public health. The great Van Swieten reprobated the use of soap, on similar grounds.

Bacon, Boyle, and Locke, were, themselves, instances of superstition, even with regard to ordinary things : this fact is undeniable. Admitting, however, that every thing here enumerated, had really happened, in the rage of a great epidemic, they would only prove, that heat, moisture, or some of the sensible qualities of the atmosphere had been in excess. At a time when terror reigns in every bosom, self-preservation must be the predominant feeling; when relation deserts re-

* In the year 1646, 200 persons were tried, condemned, and executed, for witchcraft, at the assizes for Suffolk and Essex.—*See Howel's Letters.* So late as 1699, five persons were burnt at Paisley.—*See Medical Logic.*

lation ; when the parent is unable to administer to the wants
of his offspring, or, the child to aid the parent; when the
dead lie in heaps unburied, and the infant perishes from hunger, at the cold breast of its mother ; can we wonder if domestic animals sicken and die from the mere want of food, drink,
or proper attention? Canary-birds will die, with blood at
their bills, from common diseases, brought on by common
causes, as want of drink.

Unless wild animals died in as great proportion, no inferences can be drawn in proof of atmospheric causes. Pregnant women miscarry from being relaxed by a long course of
hot weather ; but they do so, likewise, from terror ; grief for
the loss of a relation ; fatigue, or want of sleep in attending
one. During great sickness they must be called upon to per-
form more than ordinary labour.

When people wear sheets instead of shoes ; when they are
covered with blankets instead of clothes, and use spoons instead of knives or forks, is it surprising that leather gets
mouldy, that clothes moth in the chest, and iron or steel cor-
rodes ? When out of use, and therefore too long kept, will
not beef get putrid, cheese decay, butter turn rancid, milk
get sour? May not all the above things happen under such
circumstances in ordinary seasons ? If this be allowed, it
cannot be difficult to account for the rest. As flies and other
insects are attracted in prodigious numbers to any spot where
food abounds, so they, like other animals, multiply and increase under favourable circumstances. Fewer persons being astir to disturb them, the myriads that exist in great
epidemics is readily accounted for. When frogs are not
pelted by children near a large town, they, too, must breed
faster and become more audacious. When accumulation of
putrid smells, and accumulation of flies and other insects,
attract crows, magpies, and birds of prey in greater numbers
to the neighbourhood, especially at a time when every thing
around is quiet and has a deserted aspect, then sparrows,
robins, and other small birds, will be glad to decamp.

In this way we explain many of the phenomena that have been noticed by authors, as proofs of the existence of a mysterious agency in epidemic diseases. At the same time, we are well aware that we shall be ranked among common observers by all those who are above making common observations. We shall be contented to remain in this humble rank; but, at the same time, we must do ourselves the justice to deny, that the observations we have made are common; for we know of no author on epidemic diseases who has given them due consideration. The phenomena above enumerated are no more entitled to the important inferences attempted to be drawn from them, than a hundred other occurrences which are every day passing around us. There is nothing more surprising in a good breeding season for frogs, than a favourable one for lambs or turnips. Magpies hovering about a house have, in all ages, been considered a bad omen for the sick it contained : the putrid smell arising from a single patient will attract them. The carcase of a single horse first attracts flies and insects, then carrion-crows, or birds of prey. Sparrows and robins, which, in time of snow, jump into barns and outhouses from the want of food out of doors, will nevertheless decamp from the larger birds, when collected. Sharks have been observed to follow ships at sea in calm weather ; as then, the face of the ocean being unruffled, things thrown overboard float in the tract of the vessel. Gulls assemble round one at anchor after every meal taken on board; the bread-dust and other refuse being consigned to the deep at these hours attract a number of small fish on which these birds subsist. Fishermen will fill their nets with small fish to-day, to-morrow not a single one will appear, but large fish.; to the appearance of which they attribute the departure of the smaller. To be sure, sailors and fishermen are but common observers, alike unacquainted with the organic adjustments of the earth, and the mineralogical arrangements in the bottom of the ocean.

Hitherto we have confined our observations chiefly to the

E

rise and first progress of an epidemic, and endeavoured to explain why sailors and other strangers are first attacked; why, when seized, they suffer more than natives of the place; why natives having first intercourse with them are early infected; why lodging-houses, which are generally situated near the shipping are so often contaminated; why a contagious disease sometimes breaks out in different quarters of a town about the same time, without apparent communication; why it is so difficult to trace contagion from place to place; why relations, though living at a short distance from each other, are more likely to be taken ill than persons not related; why the first appearance of epidemics have so frequently been dated at the arrival of a fleet; how a ship, the crew of which has been healthy during the voyage, may yet import contagion; how to judge the momentous question of importation by ships; why epidemic diseases are occasionally irregular, even capricious and whimsical, in their course and mode of procedure; and, lastly, why they are connected with a number of unusual appearances, and which are, at first sight, apparently inexplicable on common principles. On the other hand, we ask, will any atmospheric cause account for the rise, progress, and decline of the plague of West Barbary, or the epidemic yellow fever of Cadiz and Gibraltar, soon to be described?

The after-progress and decline of epidemics seem likewise to admit of explanation.

When an epidemic plague has arrived at its height, it begins to languish, though the contagion be a million times greater in quantity than at the beginning. This is explained from—

1st, A number of persons not being susceptible, and many of those who are having fled from the place:

2d, Those who are susceptible either having died or gone through the disease:

3d, Even those who have not gone through it have become, by habit, to a considerable degree hardened against the influence of contagion:

4th, The means of prevention being better understood, they are more promptly and regularly put in practice :

5th, The people last attacked are generally those who have been least susceptible from the beginning; they have, therefore, the disease in a milder, often in an imperfect form, consequently the matter derived from them is less in quantity, and also deteriorated in quality.

6th. Where the systems through which the matter has passed happen to have been those pre-occupied with other diseases, incompatible in some measure with the prevailing disorder, the contagion will run a greater risk; but it will become deteriorated, merely by being transmitted through a number of persons of different constitutions in health.

7th. The season least favourable to the influence of the contagion having arrived.

We deem it necessary further to illustrate each of the above with examples and proof.

SUSCEPTIBILITY.—1st. *The human body is not always susceptible of contagion, nor is it always alike so to any external impression.*

As some external impressions act more uniformly the same on different constitutions than on others, so some of the contagions affect a greater number of persons in the same way than others ; all of them, however, agree in sparing a certain proportion of individuals exposed to their influence. They all, too, agree in affecting the same individuals more at one time than at another.

The skin, lungs, and stomach are the great channels through which noxious influences are received. These organs vary much in their susceptibility to external impressions in different persons, and in the same individual at different times. Of the three, however, the first differs most ; for instance, we know of no country where the natives possess striking peculiarities in their lungs or stomach, but the skin, in the people of whole nations, differs in colour, texture, and function.

E 2

The human body becomes blunted or insusceptible to certain external influences in different ways ; as by habit, disease, age, and peculiarity of constitution, called idiosyncrasy. The last only continues for life; the others, during the continuance of their causes.

Insusceptibility arising from habit will be afterwards noticed.

Particular diseases, especially those which violently affect the nervous system, confer a temporary insusceptibility to certain influences. Thus, a maniac during his paroxysm of madness, is often insensible to hunger, thirst, and cold, which would prove fatal to others ; yet this power of resisting them is instantly lost by a return to health. In lock-jaw, a similar thing takes place; the patient, though in sound mind, is able to resist doses of wine, opium, ardent spirits, and mercury during the disease, which would prove fatal to him in other diseases, or in health.

Susceptibility to external influences is generally greater in infancy. An infant has been thrown into convulsions by being exposed for a short time to the fumes arising from a single cask of spirits kept in the bar of a public-house ; yet infants bear calomel well, and instances are on record, where they have resisted contagion almost universally : nay, where they have been found alive at the breasts of their mothers, when they themselves have fallen victims to disease, to hunger, or to cold. The sweating sickness was perhaps more remarkable for sparing certain individuals, while it proved fatal to others, than any other contagious epidemical disease on record. Even the natives of certain countries, according to account, were not so liable to it as those of others. This extraordinary disease was engendered by the wretched state of the army brought to England by Henry the Seventh, previous to the battle of Bosworth. It first appeared upon its landing at Milford Haven in 1485, and it soon spread to London, where it raged from the beginning of August, to the end of October. It afterwards appeared four times in

England at unequal intervals, viz. in 1506, 1617, 1528, and last in 1551. The summer season was always the period of its commencement, and it continued from three to five months.

The violence of the attack in individuals affected, was over in fifteen hours ; but the patient was not considered secure till the expiration of twenty-four hours. Hence, the fever which was accompanied with violent perspiration, was called an Ephemera, and, as it was confined to one country, Ephemera Britannica. The numbers carried off by it were very great. In the town of Shrewsbury, where Caius, who wrote a history of the disease resided, 960 died in a few days. Here then is a noted instance of a violent epidemic, spreading by a contagion engendered by causes not similar to their effects.

Except in its form, it possessed all the characteristics of other great epidemics; it came only at distant and uncertain periods ; it shewed a partiality for Summer, like plague, yellow fever, small-pox, in certain countries, and like them it was not confined to particular localities, nor could any difference be observed in the seasons of those years to which alone it was confined : it respected, like other epidemics, certain individuals, and certain classes of society, though it differed in selecting the higher ranks. Those most liable were persons in high health, of middle age, and of better rank and condition ; children, poor and old people were less subject to its influence.—Vide *Willan, Cut. Dis.; Coxe, Med. Mus.; Edin. Med. Journal*, vol. iv. ; *Blane's Medical Logic, &c.*

The next epidemical disease, in point of singularity in its propensities and attachments, is yellow fever. The greater exemption of Negroes in the West Indies, and in North America, has attracted the notice of physicians, by many of whom it has been adduced as a proof, that yellow fever in those countries is not contagious, but arises from climate and unhealthy locality.

This doctrine has no analogy in its favour. The natives of

every climate under the sun are liable to the influence of unhealthy locality, when suddenly exposed. Natives of Holland, brought from a healthy spot of their own country, would fall sick in the island of Walcheren. In the proper seasons, even the inhabitants of this island suffer. So do people brought from the high or dry districts of England, when exposed to the Fens of Essex and Lincoln. In what country does not exactly the same thing happen. We know of no peculiarities either of lungs or stomach enjoyed by natives of certain countries, or certain districts of country, that could possibly confer such exemption.

The Negroes of the West Indies are not all born there. None of them are descended from the aborigines. On the contrary, the great proportion have been suddenly removed from the dry and sandy soil of Africa, where they were, perhaps, the most healthy people in existence. How then could they be expected to resist the baneful influence of the marshes of the West Indies on sudden exposure—a country in many respects so different from the one from which they were removed, and to which alone they had been accustomed. Such must be the reflections of every one who impartially considers the subject. Let us examine the facts.

Dr. Linning was one of the first writers who observes the exemption of Negroes. In the yellow fever of South Carolina, he says he knew of no instance of the disease amongst them, though they were equally subject as white people to bilious fever.

How is this to be accounted for? **Dr. L.** says, the yellow fever of South Carolina was contagious; yet Negroes escaped it. On the other hand, bilious fever is not contagious, but a disease arising from climate and unhealthy locality; yet they suffered in *common with white people*. According to Mr. Shower's letter before given, the Negroes in Sierra Leone suffered from marsh fever so late as the year 1826, or forty years after their importation into that colony, although Dr.

Bancroft, at p. 275, only mentions their liability, as depending on their sudden removal from colder climates.

Do we know of any mode by which Negroes could escape exposure to any atmospheric agent? To this question our answer must be in the negative. Every one residing in an unhealthy spot, must necessarily breathe the air of that place. Do we know of any mode by which persons may escape exposure to contagion in a sickly country? Our answer to this question must be, yes; for we can furnish a thousand proofs of the fact. We are led, therefore, to inquire what are the peculiarities observable in Negroes, by which they could expect exemption occasionally from a contagious disease. 1st. The skin of Negroes is somewhat different from that of white people, both in texture and function, consequently they are better secured against absorption, and less sensible to external impression. 2d. A great proportion of them wear no clothes, or at least clothes capable of becoming impregnated with human effluvia. 3d. They are a people by themselves, and of course they have less connexion with the white people, among whom the disease has been introduced. 4th. They live more in the country, and labour chiefly in the open air; a circumstance which puts them in the same relation with the shepherds and peasants in other countries. Take away these differences in their mode of life; remove the cocoa-nut oil from their surface; soften their skins, by covering them with woollen or cotton clothes for some time in a colder climate; give them a soft bed to sleep upon, instead of a bare mat; wash away their unctuous perspiration; bring them from the country into large crowded towns, where contagions most abound, and expose them to the same intercourse and communication as white people, then the result would be very different. Accordingly, when Dr. Rush, on account of the supposed insusceptibility, applied to the African Society to send Negro nurses to the sick in the great epidemic yellow fever of Philadelphia, in 1793, it was not long before they were attacked. They took the disease *in common with white people,* and many of them died of it. " A large number," says he, " were my patients. It was milder in them."

Numerous other authors have noticed the exemptions of Negroes, without referring to the peculiarities on which it seems to depend. Many others, however, among whom is Dr. Bancroft, record facts of their being affected in common with white people, when placed under similar circumstances, in cold or temperate climates. " In the fever of Philadelphia," observes Dr. Drysdale, " though they took the disease, they were less endangered, both *from their manner of living,* and from being less injured by the common exciting causes." Moseley has remarked, that among other persons, they who did not perspire freely were most subject to yellow fever. Negroes are seldom liable to this defect; their colour tends to preserve their health in situations, and under circumstances, that would prove fatal to white people ; the black ivory with which Nature has invested them, incontrovertibly preserves an unconfined discharge of perspiration, even under the influence of powerful opposers of perspiration. The design obviously indicates the forming hand of an indulgent and omnipotent Father of the Universe.

The true Negroes of Senaar, the hottest country in the world, are of a jet black complexion, and owing to the great evaporation from their surfaces, are two degrees cooler than Europeans. Wilson, in his Essay on Climate, ascribes to their food, the exemption of Negroes.—Vide *Philad. Med. Mus.* vol. i, pp. 38-9; *Phil. Trans.* 1804, *on the Nature of Heat; also, Professor Leslie's Experiments.* Dr. Currie has noticed the more unctuous, less easily dissipated, more pungent and stimulating qualities of the perspiration in the Negroes ; also the practice of oiling and anointing the skin, common amongst all savages, and some other nations. The good effects of such a state of skin, in preventing the absorption of contagion, cannot be doubted. " It has been supposed," says Dr. Bancroft in his Essay on Yellow Fever, " by

Orræus Pugnet and others, *with some probability*, that the transpiration through the skin may hinder the absorption of pestilential contagion, and even wash it out from the pores. They, therefore, recommended exercise for this purpose. Desgennettes, chief physician to the French army in Egypt, after his visits to the pest-house, always mounted his horse, and rode till he was in a profuse perspiration, with this view. —Vide *Desgennettes*, p. 90."—*Bancroft*, p. 587.

If the perspirable matter of the European could be expected to have this effect, with gross matter of plague applied to the skin by actual touch, what would be the effects of the perspiration of the Negro on the impalpable volatile and more easily dissipated contagion of yellow fever, in climates much hotter, *and where the naked surface is exposed to the air at the same time.* Yet Dr. Bancroft has overlooked this in yellow fever altogether.

It is probable that the subtle contagion of yellow fever is seldom in such a concentrated form as to affect persons exposed, through the medium of the air entering the lungs or stomach, in hot climates. The excessive heat of those climates in which it occurs, and to which it is exclusively confined, naturally suggests, at all times, the necessity of a free ventilation. To ensure this more effectually, the houses have a profusion of doors and windows, so placed as to catch every breeze. Few of the windows in the houses of the West Indies are furnished with glass, but blinds to admit the fresh air, without the sun's heat. In general they are very large, reaching down to the floor of each apartment of the house; and, as they are made to open, they are used as doors as well as windows. On these accounts, the air in the apartments, which are very large, and high in the ceilings, is oftener renewed than that in the houses of colder climates. At night in particular, the current of air passing through them is so strong, as to require protecting shades to the lamps or candles. " It is impossible," says Dr. Jackson, " to refuse assent to the inference, that there is something in the tempe-

rature of tropical climates, in the thorough ventilation of tropical houses, in the routine of personal cleanliness that
usually obtains among the troops in hot countries, which
strongly counteracts the propagation of certain forms of contagious diseases."—Vol. i, p. 32. In climates like that of
North America and Spain, the houses are somewhat differently furnished. Here, it being as necessary to keep them
warm in Winter, as it is to keep them cool in Summer, they
cannot be fitted for both purposes; and, as there is a greater
proportion of towns, many of which are wretchedly built,
the bad effects of crowding and imperfect ventilation must
be more felt; of course, the danger to Negroes, accustomed to the country air, greater. The peculiarities of the
skin of the Negro can only secure him against the absorption of contagion through its pores; but we have given
reasons why he is less liable to receive it by the other two
channels, while he lives only in a tropical climate. Some
writers of respectability, have indeed, been inclined to doubt
whether the matter of contagion is ever taken in by the skin,
excepting in parts where the cuticle or scarf-skin has been
abraded. This opinion, however, is contradicted by too
many facts to be entitled to much attention. We know, for
instance, that the plague is only infectious by actual contact,
yet that millions have been seized with this disease, without
having received it by the stomach *or broken scarf-skin*, is
perfectly evident. If it could have been received in breathing the air of an apartment, how does it in every case require
touch. Abrasion of the cuticle or scarf-skin will, however,
facilitate the absorption of contagion, by the skin.

May not this last fact partly account for the greater liability of Europeans to contagious diseases in hot climates?
Those who have never experienced the distress arising from
the thickly-set and often universally diffused eruption on the
skin, called "prickly heat," and the many sleepless and
feverish nights occasioned by the bites of bugs, gnats, musquitoes, centipedes, &c. in those climates, may smile at this

idea. What with these pests and scratching, we have seen parts of the body nearly reduced to a raw surface, and even producing slight fever. We have likewise witnessed serious and even fatal consequences, from the sudden suppression of prickly heat. If absorption of contagion by the skin be allowed, will not a broken state of it facilitate that process? Nor are the face and hands free from eruption. On the delicate complexion of an European lady, its ravages are truly frightful.

Natives of hot climates are not troubled with any pests of this kind. " The musquitoes and other insects," Mr. Jackson observes, " attack strangers with great keenness, biting them and sucking their blood in a most distressing manner. The thick skins of the Arabs, *exposed daily to the scorching heat of the sun,* are impregnable to their bite, otherwise they would not be able to exist."—Vide *Jackson's Morocco.*

We have many instances in our own country of a similar kind. By handling hot iron more frequently, the skin of a blacksmith's palms and fingers become thickened and insensible to heat, much more so to touch. By the practice of walking without shoes, the Scotch and Irish peasants are enabled to pass over the roughest ground without inconvenience; and the naked savage will penetrate a jungle or forest, that would appal the clothed European.

The perspiration differs more in different climates than has generally been supposed. Few persons who like to try it, will make a mistake between the smell of a Negro and that of a European or native of a cool or temperate region. That the perspiration even of the European becomes changed by residence in a hot climate, can as little be doubted. It may be partly owing to this cause, that musquitoes and other insects seldom make a mistake in selecting for their prey the bodies of the newly-arrived, in preference to those who have resided some time in a hot climate. It is probable, that the juices become less sweet; and, being partly mixed with bile, are less palatable to those insects. One thing cannot be doubted, the prickly heat declines by residence, and in proportion as a free and regular perspiration is established. May not these differences partly account for the less susceptibility of Europeans, who have resided some time in a hot climate, to the contagion of yellow fever? That Negroes should have the disease in a milder form is nothing more remarkable, than that persons living on a vegetable diet, and leading a temperate life, should run less risk of inflammation, gout, or apoplexy, than those who live on rich animal food, drink wine and spirits, and bid defiance to every known law of Nature. Having thus considered the much-agitated subject of the less liability of Negroes to yellow fever, in its different bearings, we shall leave our readers to determine, whether the important fact depends entirely on climate, or whether the circumstances we have noticed are worthy of consideration.

Moseley, who denies contagion in plague, as well as of yellow fever, observes of the latter—" How a climate should foster a disease, and a contagious one, and the natives of that climate be exempted from it, I cannot comprehend." But had this excellent writer paid sufficient attention to the real causes of contagious diseases in every climate, viz. the state and condition of mankind, he would have had a satisfactory solution of this difficulty. In what country do not natives of the climate suffer less from a contagious disease *of their own climate than strangers*, brought from countries where the disease is unknown? " The race we must consider (says Dr. Robertson) as the natives of these colonies, (West-Indian) are the Mulattoes and people of colour, descended from the connexion between the Europeans and Africans; and there certainly does not exist any proof that this class of men are more exempted from the endemical or epidemical diseases of their country, than what takes place amongst the natives of any other climate."—*On the Natural History of the Atmosphere*, vol. ii.

The view here taken of the causes of the less susceptibility

of Negroes to the contagion of yellow fever is further confirmed
by what happens in plague. The very learned and distinguished author, Dr. Parr, observes, that " plague may still be
pronounced *eminently* infectious; small-pox, measles, yellow
fever, the ulcerated throat, scarlatina, the catarrhus epide-
micus, and hooping-cough are probably so *in a decreasing
ratio, according to the order.''—Art. Contagio.* Yet plague,
the first on the list of contagions, has been observed, in all
ages, to respect some individuals more than others.

According to Assilini—" Of the inhabitants of Jaffa, who
perished by the plague, a great number were infants, very few
women, some men, *almost all strangers.* In general, the
temperament and constitution of body, *state of the fluids,* age
and sex of the patient, the season, the air, the winds, situation, the fear of death, and all the affections of the mind,
modified this disease more or less; persons of a *full habit,*
infants with *a fair skin* and flaxen hair, young people of a
sanguine temperament and irritable fibres, were more liable to
the disease than those *advanced in years,* or of a dry *bilious*
habit." Assilini was so confident of the non-liability of some
persons to plague, that he encouraged a French merchant of
Jaffa, who, in consequence of the contagion, thought himself
gone, on the grounds that he considered his temperament " *a
complete protection* from the disease."—*P.* 32.

Exemptions from epidemical diseases are found recorded in
the history of every pestilential disorder. Mercurialis observed, in a plague, which was more prevalent in Pavia than
any where else, the indolent, luxurious, debauched, and men
servants were most liable to be affected. In the great plague
of London, a prodigious proportion of those who died were
servants. This fact is accounted for, merely by their having
greater intercourse, by going messages, &c. into the most
public places. Pliny thought *old people not so liable* to
plague. Some German authors mention they saw several infants suckling nurses ill of the plague, yet escaped; several
nurses died of the disease, the infants remaining unhurt.

The external use of oil, however, furnishes the best illustration of the causes of exemption, in Negroes, from contagion; oil-frictions to the skin having been found an effectual
security against the absorption of plague. George Baldwin,
Esq. formerly Consul General in Egypt, has inserted an interesting article on this subject in Duncan's Annals of Medicine for 1797. That gentleman states that, among upwards
of a million of inhabitants carried off by the plague in Upper
and Lower Egypt, during four years, he could not hear of a
single instance of an oilman, or dealer in oil, suffering from
this terrible disease. He likewise mentions, that there is no
instance of a person rubbing a patient having taken the infection. The following quotation from Mr. Jackson serves
further to illustrate the same subject.

" In the Kingdom of Tunis, the people usually employed
as coolies, or porters, are in general natives of Gereed, or the
Country of Dates, about 300 miles from the sea-coast. Their
dress is, in general, a wide woollen coat, its natural colour,
with short wide sleeves over, wrapping around the body, and
tied round the waist with a circular band; they never wear a
shirt, and seldom have either trowsers, shoes, or stockings;
they have always a scarlet woollen cap upon the head, and
sometimes a coarse white turban. Those coolies that are
employed in the oil-stores seldom eat any thing but bread and
oil; they smear themselves all over with oil, and their coat is
always well soaked with it. Though the plague frequently
rages at Tunis in the most frightful manner, destroying many
thousands of the inhabitants, yet there was never known an
instance of any of these coolies, who work in the oil-stores,
ever being in the least affected by it. In the Summer, it is
customary for these coolies to sleep in the streets upon the
bare ground. We have frequently seen, in the night, scorpions
and other venomous reptiles running about them in great
numbers, yet we never heard of a single instance where the
coolies were ever injured by them; nor do the musquitoes,
which are always very troublesome to other people in hot cli-

mates, ever molest these people, though their face, hands, and arms, from their elbows, are exposed, as also their legs and feet : any other people being so much exposed, would be nearly destroyed by the musquitoes.

" In Tunis, when any person is stung by a scorpion, or any other venomous reptile, they immediately scarify the part with the knife, and rub in olive oil as quick as possible, which arrests the progress of the venom. If oil is not applied in a few minutes, death is inevitable, particularly from the sting of a scorpion. Those in the kingdom of Tunis are the most venomous in the world.

" The strength and agility of these coolies and porters are almost incredible. Having a great many ships to load, we employed several of these people, and have frequently seen one of them carry a load upon his back which weighed half a ton English weight, a distance of thirty or forty yards."— *Reflections on the Commerce of the Mediterranean.*

The French sçavans in Egypt say that, in one year, in which the plague carried off a million of people in Egypt, there was no instance of an oil-porter being attacked by it. —*See Memoirs Relative to Egypt, &c.* During the great plague in London, the tallow-chandlers enjoyed, it is said, a similar exemption. According to Dr. Witman, the merchants of Cairo positively affirm, that the oil-sellers, water-carriers, and tanners are not subject to plague. Captain Franklin has stated, on the authority of a Mr. Thornton, a respectable merchant of Constantinople, that the same exemption is enjoyed by the oil-sellers in that city, and that wearing shirts dipped in oil had been found useful in preventing the disease. Mr. Eton, in his survey of the Turkish Empire, says the plague is unknown to those nations who are accustomed to rub their bodies with oil. M. Assilini, who was a medical officer in the French army in Egypt, makes likewise a favourable report of oil frictions in plague, as being generally followed *by copious sweatings,* to which he attributes their power of prevention. Mr. Jackson recommended the practice to several Jews and Mussulmen during the plague of West Barbary ; and without any instance of its failure, when daily persevered in, even after infection had manifested itself. Sir James M'Grigor mentions a similar fact. He observed that the men who were employed in applying oily frictions to the camels for some epidemy affecting them, escaped the plague.—*Medical Sketches.* Dr. Mitchell quotes a similar exemption from pestilential fever, or the yellow fever of Philadelphia in 1793, enjoyed by the tallow-chandlers of that city; and by those of New York in 1795-6. It is probable that friction, with oily and unctuous substances on the skin, acts beneficially in preventing the absorption of contagious matter, in three different ways. 1st. By filling up the mouths of the extreme vessels, and thereby hindering it entering the body. 2nd. By diluting the matter on the surface, or washing it away. 3d. By its relaxing the pores, it excites a free discharge of perspiration at the same time. In promoting sweat, the friction itself must be taken into account. The exemption of water-carriers can only be explained on the second principle here mentioned ; namely, by diluting it, or removing it altogether from the hands or places to which it has been applied. As the hands are more exposed than other parts of the body to contagion, tallow-chandlers might be rendered pretty secure on the same principles. In tanners, who have their hands and arms exposed to the action of the air and cold water, those parts become thickened, independent of the tanning powers of the astringent matters in which they are often immersed. It is probable that, by such means, the parts exposed become hardened, and to a certain degree insensible to external impressions, like the skin of the Negro, by exposure to the weather. A nurse's nipples, when so tender that they can scarcely be touched, or admit of the child's suckling, may be rendered hard and more insensible by an infusion of oak-bark, such as tanners use in their trade.

A remarkable instance of exemption from yellow fever, is mentioned by Sir James Fellowes. " During the yellow fever," of 1800, at Xeres, says he, " there were thirty-eight persons, men and women, including nine children, daily employed about the tan-vats ; that two of the men were sent every morning to market, to provide for the rest of the party, whilst the disorder was carrying off 180 to 250 a day in the towns, yet neither the two workmen, nor any of the others, or their families within the building, ever had the slightest symptoms of the disease."

" The same exemption was observed during the epidemic of 1804. As this tan-yard was situated to the eastward of the town, did the east winds, which were said to prevail, and blowing in that direction towards the town, contribute to its salubrity, or was it owing to the people living within the building being constantly surrounded by the tan-vats ? That it more probably arose from the latter cause, appears from this fact, that the nearest building to the tan-yard, about *forty yards* to the rear, (East we presume,) was a barrack, in which a part of the regiment of Spanish carabiniers were quartered at the same time, and several of the soldiers were taken ill there, and sent to the hospital at the other end of the town."—*On Yellow Fever*, pp. 441-2-3.

The men going to market, as here stated, could not but be exposed to every atmospheric cause of yellow fever. . If, during their intercourse, they handled infected articles, we have little doubt but they would be less susceptible, on the principles already explained. Frictions with oil do not seem to have received a full trial as a preventive of the yellow fever in Spain. By some a favourable report of a few trials has been given; but Sir J. Fellowes and Arejula doubt the truth of these reports. We would here observe the great difference between the state of society in the close streets and crowded towns of Spain, a country much colder, and that in the West Indies. Oil frictions can never prevent a concentrated dose of the poison from entering the lungs and stomach.

Oil has been used in the cure of plague, as well as in the

F

prevention. Assilini mentions its success in the hospital at Smyrna, where 250 persons were received in five years, and all who were treated in this way recovered.—P. 47.

Dr. Hufeland thought oil was only useful in the cure of plague when *a great perspiration* ensued. Its use amongst the Égyptians, in pestilential fevers, is mentioned by Alpinus. As the external application of oil to the skin was practised to a vast extent amongst the ancients, their greater exemption from cutaneous diseases in general, and from some of our contagious distempers, is the more readily accounted for.

Baron Larrey states that, before the French army left Syria, a great number of the soldiers were attacked with plague ; yet it seldom seized the wounded men, and scarcely an instance occurred of any one being affected by it whilst their wounds were in *a state of suppuration,* nor until they healed up. Artificial blisters and issues have, therefore, been recommended as preventives.

Small-pox is second on the list of Dr. Parr, in point of its powers of infecting; yet some constitutions are not susceptible to the disease in any form. Others do not receive it at one time, however freely exposed to its contagion, *even though repeatedly inoculated,* and yet receive it afterwards, by merely approaching the sick. Dr. Huxham, in his Treatise on Fevers, &c., says, " I know an old nurse, and one apothecary, who, for many years attended persons, and a great number too, in the small-pox, and yet never had it; nay, *many* that have industriously endeavoured to catch the infection, by frequenting the chambers of the sick, have done it *without effect ;* and yet, some of those persons, some months or years after, have been seized with the small-pox." " Laws," says Hennen, " which we can never develop, govern the susceptibility to variolous contagion ; and, it is highly probable, as has been observed by the ingenious Jenner, that the susceptibility to receive it, always remains through life, *but under various modifications or gradations,* from that point where it passes silently and imperceptibly through the constitution (as is frequently the case with cow-pox), up to that where it appears in a confluent state, and with such violence as to destroy life."—*See Ed. Med. Journ.* vol. 14.

Non-susceptibility to small-pox has even been observed in whole communities. " I have sometimes observed," says Van Swieten, " large towns to be free from small-pox, whilst it raged epidemically in the neighbouring villages; and, on the contrary, some large towns *universally* visited by the complaint, *whilst the villages in the neighbourhood remained in health,* though the inhabitants of both *mixed daily with each other."* He carried two patients of his into a large town, without propagating the contagion there ; and he adds, "many respectable physicians have told me the same thing."

" The small-pox," says Sir John Pringle, " being carried into a camp by some new-raised recruits, quickly disappeared, without becoming general, although it is notorious that other camp diseases are but too apt to spread themselves."

When Sir James M'Grigor was at Bombay, the small-pox was raging in the houses contiguous to the barracks, yet not one adult or child was affected by it. The late Dr. Otter mentions, in a letter to Dr. Haygarth, " that we have frequently inoculated, at Geneva, a great number of children, in the years during which small-pox was not epidemic; those children have gone out every day, even after the eruption had broken out; they have been in the streets and in the public walks ; they have communicated freely with other children susceptible of the infection; and not only the small-pox did not spread, but there did not occur, to my knowledge, any distinct instance of the communication of the disease from one individual to another in the streets or promenades."

So late as the end of the Summer, 1818, the small-pox committed great ravages in Norwich, an event which cannot surprize any one who is acquainted with the loose state of our laws regarding contagion, and the prejudices existing against vaccination. The disease was introduced by a girl arrived from York, who had caught it on the road.

" In January, 1819, (says Mr. Cross*) a druggist inoculated three children, thereby helping to keep up the contagion brought to the city, as stated, in the end of the previous Summer.

" The town of Norwich had been nearly or entirely free from small-pox from 1805 till 1807; again, from 1807 till 1813; again, from 1813 till the period above alluded to. In February, 1819, the disease got into one of the large charity schools—from this it extended to all parts of the city, and laid the foundation," adds Mr. Cross, "*for the most extensive destruction of human life* that has ever, I believe, taken place in Norwich, in the same space of time, from any other cause than the plague."

In this year, 500 *persons* died within the bills of mortality, which do not include several hamlets in the immediate neighbourhood, where it also prevailed. Mr. C. calculates, from various sources, that one in six who were affected died, and that considerably above 3000 *individuals, or about one-tenth* of the whole population of Norwich, had the disease.

It appeared in this epidemic, as is usual, that a certain proportion of persons, although *freely exposed* and unprotected, *resisted the contagion.* Mr. Cross kept a register of the effects produced by the contagion in 112 families, comprising 603 persons, into which it was introduced. In these families, 297, or nearly one-half, had had small-pox before, and escaped; 91 had been vaccinated and escaped, excepting *three,* who had a mild disease; 200, who were unprotected, took small-pox, and 15, though unprotected, escaped; of which number, *ten had been likewise exposed to the contagion before with impunity.*

" The small-pox occurred, in several instances, in adults, who had, *at various times* before, resisted intimate and continued exposure to its contagion. A man who believed himself to have had the disease, lived for twelve years as a nurse in the establishment for the reception of inoculated patients, near

* On the Variolous Epidemic of Norwich.

Norwich, continually waiting on the patients who were under-going the disease, and at the end of that time he caught the small-pox, of which he died." Had such a mode of medical enquiry as that adopted by Mr. Cross been commenced as early as the days of Sydenham, humanity would not now have to deplore the fate of countless thousands who have, since his time, fallen victims to this terrible disease.

Our limits will not permit us to pursue the subject of sus-ceptibility further. These instances of exemption from conta-gious diseases of the most formidable kind, are not singular; volumes might be filled with proof of the same kind, yet what would it serve to shew? Certainly not that plague, small-pox, and yellow fever are not contagious diseases; but merely that no malady is alike infectious at all times and under every circumstance. Mr. Hunter mentions an instance of twenty persons being bitten by a mad dog, yet only one of them took hydrophobia. Would we argue, from the circumstance of nineteen persons escaping, that the twentieth had not hydro-phobia, or that this distemper was not infectious?

The first time that yellow fever appeared in Gibraltar, only 28 persons escaped it out of the whole civil population, amounting to fourteen thousand. Would we argue from the fact, that every individual who had been attacked with the disease the first time escaped it on a another visit, (viz. 3,800 out of 7,370) that yellow fever is not contagious? Yet it is astonishing to reflect how much this negative evidence has influenced the minds of medical men. The most trifling and casual change in the features of a disease, the simultaneous or even previous occurrence of other diseases in men or in cattle, the slightest deviation in the rise and progress of the contagion at one time from another, its observing laws some-what different from those which govern other contagions, or the most ordinary appearances of weather, are circumstances which have all been eagerly laid hold of, and greatly exagge-rated, with a view to assist and prop up this lame negative evidence. The occurrence of any two of the above circum-

-stances, during an epidemic, is deemed quite sufficient to
stamp its ·character, and overturn the experience of ages;
whilst differences in point of exposure to contagion, and the
susceptibility of those exposed, are generally left out of view.
A smaller proportion of persons exposed to the infection
will have hydrophobia, than, perhaps, any other contagion,
and the disease will be much longer of manifesting itself in
those who take it. Some authors compute that only *one* in
sixteen, bitten by a rabid animal, will take the disease ; and
most agree that it may remain dormant in the system for
years before infection is certain. The important circumstance of the bite, however, is not soon forgotten ; hence no
one doubts that canine madness is infectious. In cases of
infection from other diseases, they have nothing to speak
home to the feelings; they, therefore, proceed on the erroneous principle, that because a man does not know when and
where he has been bitten, he is not bitten at all.

ATTACKS THE SAME PERSON ONLY ONCE.—2d. *The same
Individual is not so liable to be affected a second Time with
acute or febrile Contagious Diseases.*

With regard to small-pox, cow-pox, chicken-pox, measles,
scarlet fever, hooping-cough, and mumps, this law of contagion cannot be doubted. In yellow fever, plague, and typhus
fever it is likewise certain, though, perhaps, instances of a
second attack are oftener observed in the latter diseases.

" Small-pox has been considered by many, a disease in
which after susceptibility is wholly destroyed. This, however, is a very great mistake. The occurrence of small-
pox for the second time in the same person, which was doubted
by some, and held to be quite marvellous by almost all, has
been shewn, by the accurate observations and learned researches of Dr. Hennen and by the more extended and la-
borious inquiries of Dr. Thomson, to be, though a rare, by
no means an anomalous event."—*Edin. Med. Journ.* vol. xvi.
The paper of Dr. Hennen here alluded to, will be found in

the fourteenth volume of this excellent work. " Dr. Bateman," says Dr. H., " has lately given us two unequivocal cases of the same kind, in the second volume of the Medico-Chirurgical Transactions, and has referred to some others; among them some fatal cases. But for the satisfaction of those who may wish to consult and analyse many more authors, I give, in a note, a very long catalogue, the basis of which is formed from the ' Literaturæ Medica Digesta' of the learned and industrious Plouquet, to which I have added a few recent authorities. It is probable that others are to be found on record, and that many, since the time of Rhases, have escaped all observations whatever, or, in the unbounded confidence of practitioners to the universality of the law, that the disease can be taken but once, have been set down as cases of aggravated or confluent varicella," (chicken-pox).

The instances of a second attack of small-pox, mentioned by Professor Dr. John Thomson, of Edinburgh, may be seen in his Letter to Sir James M'Grigor, published in 1820. We have been informed of some cases of this kind, which took place on board His Majesty's ships Talbot and Rose, at Malta; but, as our informer was not a medical man, we cannot vouch for the accuracy of his statement, nor can we give the particulars. In the Alligator, when at Halifax, several cases occurred in adults, who were absolutely pitted with the former attack, some of whom died. In the epidemic small-pox at Malta, of 1830, afterwards to be described, no less than forty-two well-attested cases of a second attack occurred out of 2691, the whole number seized up to the 31st July. Many of these cases came under our own observation. A number of examples of a second attack of measles are likewise recorded by authors. In the American Medical Repository, vol. v, a number of cases are mentioned of *spurious forms* of the disease at New York, which were found to be insufficient to protect the system from a second attack.— See also the works of Willan on the same subject. The same thing has been observed in other febrile contagions, particularly where the first attacks were in a mild or imperfect form. These exceptions, however, can never shake our confidence, or at least blind us to the general rule, which seems to be as certain, fixed, and uniform, as any other law of nature; *viz.* that the same individual is not liable to a second attack of those diseases. The law, indeed, is believed to be less evident in plague, typhus, and yellow fever; but, even in them, it is sufficiently ascertained to mark the class of diseases to which they belong.

Mr. Tully, in his history of the great plague which raged in Malta and the Ionian Islands, observes—" We are taught to believe, or at least it is a received opinion, that plague may attack the same persons more than once, during life. Now, although I am not prepared to combat that belief with proof sufficient to establish, beyond controversy, a contrary doctrine, nevertheless, I can assert, from my own experience, that, of twelve persons employed as expurgators and hospital attendants at Corfu, ten of the number had the plague at Malta, nearly *three years before,* whilst the remaining two had suffered from the disease, about *four years* previously, at Constantinople. Further, I employed four soldiers of De Rolle's regiment, who had been attacked with the plague at Corfu, as orderlies in Cephalonia; and, although the duties of all had been alike extended, those persons continued, throughout the plague, *perfectly free from disease.* There were, also, among the number of expurgators and persons employed in removing the sick and burying the dead at Cephalonia, several who had the plague *years before* at Smyrna and in other parts of Turkey; and such was the confidence of the whole of them in their immunity from the disease, that they could not be prevailed upon to have recourse to the slightest precautions whatever. *One and all escaped disease.* All our best endeavours to secure their fellow-labourers *who had never had the disease before,* too frequently proved *abortive.*"

Mr. Tully adds, " in the long intercourse I have had with

plague, and with persons who have lived many years in the Levant, I have never been able to prove the fact, of plague being capable of being communicated *a second time to the same individual, nor have I éver witnessed a single case of relapse.*" The impressions on his mind, therefore, are, that we certainly are not susceptible of plague *more than once through life.*—See pp. 236-7-8, and 40.

We have made strict inquiry at Malta, Corfu, and in different parts of Greece, and in Turkey, as to the validity of Mr. Tully's opinion, and the universal answer was, that *true* plague never attacks the same person twice during life. When the first indisposition was so slight as scarcely to confine the patient, or be certainly ascertained as plague at all, it has been followed, in many instances, with a severe and even fatal attack at a future period. On the other hand, where the first attack was pretty severe, and perfectly recognizable as true plague, it has been succeeded at another time by a slight febrile attack, accompanied with bubo in the groin ; but in no instance we have heard of, has the same individual ever gone twice through a completely formed disease, or one which run a regular and unequivocal course in both instances. Sympathetic bubo, accompanied with slight fever, is by no means a rare occurrence in the Mediterranean. They frequently arise from a slight strain, fatigue from walking, &c., and are of an irregular form, having a broad and undefined base. Although accompanied with slight fever, the tumour itself is generally indolent, and seldom comes the length of suppuration ; or, when at length it does so, suppurates partially. We have found compression, by a tight flannel bandage and linen compress, remove them with the help of opening medicines. We agree, therefore, with Mr. Tully, in thinking, that such cases as we have described, have sometimes been taken for plague. In one case we saw of this kind, the fever was of a typhoid kind, attended with raving during sleep. The tendency to these kind of buboes must be increased by plague, or any disease which is known

to affect more particularly the same glands. Dr. Bancroft
saw two cases of re-infection, or second attacks of plague in
Egypt. The patients, he adds, were, however, *but slightly
indisposed*, though each had a bubo. Dr. Buchan had a
second attack, but with only a *small carbuncle*. Dr. Rice
also had a second attack, *without either bubo or carbuncle*,
but with violent headach. " In general," says Dr. Bancroft,
" I think second attacks *are milder* than the first, though Dr.
Rice informed me, of his having seen a lad die of one."
Pugnet, p. 140, says, " When they occurred, they were oftenest in persons who had *been mildly treated* by the first
attack."—P. 599.

The exemption of persons from a second attack of plague,
was known as early as the great plague of Athens. Thucydides, who has given one of the best histories of a great
epidemic, perhaps extant, says of this plague: " But those
that recovered had much compassion, both on them that
died, and on them that lay sick, as having both known the
misery themselves, *and now no longer subject to the danger.
For the disease never took any man the second time, so as to
be mortal;* and these men both by others, were counted
happy, and they also themselves, through excess of present
joy, conceived a kind of slight hope, never to die of any
other sickness hereafter."*

This account, given by Thucydides at so remote a period,
may be regarded as a singular confirmation of what has been
stated by Tully, in the last great epidemic plague recorded.
He says, that *slight febrile* attacks were sometimes observed
in persons who had plague, *but those bore no resemblance to
the original disease.* The statement made by both, is further
confirmed by what has been generally observed in other contagious distempers.

Mr. Bryce, of Edinburgh, who had paid great attention to

* Lucretius, in his book On the Nature of Things, has given a beautiful
description of this plague.

small-pox, says :—" I believe, also, that it may be regarded as *a general rule,* that those persons who have suffered an attack of small-pox, may be considered safe against a future attack of that disease : that, from some peculiarity of constitution, however, which we cannot explain, certain persons who have suffered an attack of small-pox are liable again, on exposure to infection, to suffer *a considerable constitutional disorder."* " That the constitutional disorder thus excited is generally *more slight* than a first attack of small-pox, but that we have on record more instances of persons suffering severely, nay fatally, from what was considered to be a second attack of small-pox, than from small-pox after, what has been considered, perfect vaccination."—See *on Vaccination, Edinburgh Medical Journal,* vol. xiv.

Some confused notion of the non-liability of persons to a second attack of plague, seems to have been entertained by the people of London, in the great epidemic of 1665. The author of the Plague in London, when describing the disorderly conduct of the populace, adds—" the common people believed that *the air* was, like a person *in small-pox, not liable to be twice infected with plague."* This observation, made at a time when the air was believed to be *the only source of infection,* is certainly very remarkable, and is sufficiently corroborative of a faith in our present doctrine.

The following accurate observations of Hodges, in his account of the same plague, deserve to be mentioned.

1st. " A pestilence that is fierce and deadly in its first attack soon ceases.

2d. " The times of a pestilence, in its decrease, are in proportion to the times of its increase.

3d. " The cause of a pestilence being removed, *spent,* or extinguished, its effects immediately cease. As fire, (he adds) goes out when its fuel is wanting *or spent,* so the pestilential virulence continually wants *something* to keep it up, and no longer than it is supplied with that *necessary pabulum* will it last."—*Hodges on the Plague of London in* 1665, *pp.* 144-5.

We need not tell our readers that that *something*—that *necessary pabulum*, here mentioned as a requisite to keep up a pestilence, is human bodies susceptible of its contagion, and unprotected by any previous attack of plague.

HABIT.—3d. *The human body becomes less susceptible of contagion by frequent exposure to its influence.*

The power of habit in disarming noxious influences is not confined to contagion, but extends to many other impressions. By degrees, the dose of laudanum may be increased from 40 drops to four ounces ; yet, if the individual who takes it be gradually brought back to the original dose, or leave off taking it for some time, a large dose might prove fatal. The stomach is so irritable, as to be readily excited by passing a feather into the fauces ; yet the Indian Juggler, by habit, learns to pass a sword down the gullet into that organ. In like manner, prisoners confined in a jail contaminated with contagion, sometimes resist its influence, and remain healthy; yet, when brought out even into an open and airy court of justice for trial, they quickly infect others, who have been accustomed only to breathe a pure air. In the same way medical men, who are in the constant practice of attending fever patients in their own dirty, ill-aired, and crowded dwellings, are seldom attacked with contagious diseases, whereas the unhabituated student or nurse frequently falls a victim to the contagion of the large and better-ventilated apartment of an hospital.

We need not enlarge on this point, which, however well known by others, has not been sufficiently adverted to by medical writers. The power of habit in diminishing susceptibility has not unfrequently been wholly overlooked; as a proof of which, the fact of a greater proportion of medical attendants escaping a disease, is still held up as evidence of non-contagion. According to Procopius, none of the physicians or attendants on the sick were affected in the dreadful plague of Constantinople in 543, although it continued between two and three years. But who would contend, from a hundred such facts, that plague is not a contagious disease?

4th. *The means of prevention are better understood and more generally practised.*

In most epidemic plagues upon record, the disease had made considerable progress before its real nature was recognized, or at least generally acknowledged. The dogmatic scepticism of some, the knavery of others, and the ignorance, folly, obstinacy, and confusion of all, had to be detected and removed, by the sacrifice of countless numbers, before the public authorities or the people were convinced, either of the expediency of measures of prevention, or the best method of adopting them. Weather-wisdom, in particular, has cost the lives of millions. In some instances, the physicians differed in opinion from the magistrates, and the people from both. In no case have medical men agreed amongst themselves : the juniors in the profession, at all times anxious to court notoriety, have sometimes been too rash in dissenting from the opinions of the more experienced. " Obstinate, because untaught by experience—rash, because unacquainted with danger—headstrong, because unsubdued by disappointment," they too often impute the necessary caution of their seniors to the prejudices of early education, or to the imbecility of age. Opinions once started must be supported at all hazards; hence, the oaths of smugglers and vagabonds have been eagerly collected to contradict respectable testimony.

Need we wonder if, under such a state of things, epidemics are generally at their height before any thing like wise and efficient measures of prevention are adopted? A great deal of confusion takes place, even in cases where they are earlier put in practice. From the want of a regular system of medical police, no one knows either his post or his duty. It is like beginning to drill men for soldiers to defend a place, when the enemy have gotten possession of the town; or firemen learning for the first time to extinguish a conflagration, when every quarter of it is in flames. There is, however, this great and important difference between the cases here mentioned; in the two first the enemies are visible, whereas contagion is a hidden invader and an insidious foe.*

DETERIORATION OF MATTER.—5th and 6th. *The matter of contagion becomes deteriorated, by passing through a number of bodies, in the course of an epidemic.*

It was the opinion of the celebrated Jenner, that even the vaccine virus, although propagated only by art, became deteriorated in its quality, in consequence of passing through a succession of individuals of the human species, without recurring to the original source of the disease in the cow and horse. He has been opposed in this opinion, by Mr. Moore, in his History of Vaccination, and Professor Thomson, on the grounds, 1st. That no such deterioration has ever been observed of any other contagious disease. 2d. That the vaccine virus used at the Royal Public Dispensary, Edinburgh, and of other parts of Scotland, for a series of 18 years, still possessed all its original qualities. 3d. That recent equine matter sent down to him by Dr. Jenner, produced exactly the same appearances.—*Edin. Journ.*, vol. xvi. p. 238.

We would beg leave to remark, however, that the two last statements here made by Dr. Thomson, even if admitted as facts, (which we do not presume to dispute,) cannot be received as proof of the correctness of his first observation. Where a contagion is propagated *by art*, every circumstance

---

* It is not necessary to adduce much evidence of a fact so well known. " If (says Mr. Cross) the inhabitants of Norwich could have been made duly aware of this fact (the importance of vaccination), at the time when the disease began to spread in 1819, and had then taken the same measures to insure the protection of all who were liable to small-pox *which they actually took at a subsequent period of the epidemic,* the statements contained in the present volume are, of themselves, sufficient to shew *that they would have effectually arrested its progress.*" A similar neglect took place at Malta in the fatal epidemic of 1830.

is naturally taken due advantage of, to ensure complete success. Choice is made of the patient from whom the matter is taken, the period of the disease in him, the nature of his constitution, the state of his health at the time of taking it and through the progress of his disease, and also the state of the pustule from which it is extracted. Besides these circumstances, regard is paid to the age, health, and condition of the person to be exposed to the influence of the virus. That they have been able to keep up a proper supply of good matter at the vaccine establishment of Edinburgh for so long a period, is therefore nothing remarkable, especially when we consider the great number of patients vaccinated, and *the choice of subjects* which this number afforded. In cases of *natural propagation*, as in the usual course of a great epidemic, no such rules are observed. As the young, the healthy, and robust, in other words, the most susceptible, are first attacked in every epidemic, the matter of contagion, it is true, runs much less risk of being deteriorated : so long as the disease is confined to subjects of this kind, as it possesses *all the advantages of artificial propagation*, the virus may be expected to maintain much of its original purity. At a more advanced period of the epidemic, however, many circumstances are totally changed. Then, the old, infirm, emaciated, and sickly, become the subjects of the reigning disease ; consequently the contagion, like every other secretion, whether healthy or morbid, must be influenced by the change. The most combustible materials being now consumed, the disease may be expected to languish like a fire, when incombustible matters become involved.

By the time that an epidemic has arrived at its height, the matter of contagion, in passing through the systems of many individuals in succession, must have been applied to one subject at one period of the disorder, to another at another; and the nature of the constitutions exposed to its influence, must have been as various as the matter taken at different stages of the disease. Some persons have the disease in an imperfect form, and, in them, a spurious matter is generated. Many have their systems pre-occupied with other diseases, to a certain degree unfavourable to the prevailing distemper, while others are too feeble for their constitutions to enter into the action necessary to form a complete disease.

Such are the manifest differences between the *artificial* and *accidental* propagation of contagion. Where no regard is paid to rules, we know that neither inoculation nor vaccination will afford security against small-pox. Mr. Cross, the author before quoted, observes that, besides the interruption of the pustules by rubbing, or extracting too much ichor, numerous other causes may interfere with the progress of the vaccine pock, which may be disregarded at the time, and subsequently, in the absence of a register, forgotten; *particularly diseases pre-occupying the system* at the surface of the skin. Cleghorn (of Wirtemburgh) mentions that, in a district where scabies was so endemic that not above one in fifty was free from it, numerous cases of small-pox, both modified and regular, occurred in the vaccinated; and, on inquiry, it was found that a child with scabies had been vaccinated, *from whom ichor had been taken which produced an irregular and imperfect disease.*

An author who recently undertook an investigation of the causes of failure of vaccination in Siberia, has related that, in 1816, above 100 who had been vaccinated had small-pox, *in the same district,* and some of them died. It happened that they had all been vaccinated by *one surgeon,* who was suspended from his office as vaccinator, while an inquiry was instituted by a medical committee expressly appointed. It was ascertained that the surgeon had been in the habit of taking ichor, *as late as the tenth day,* from vesicles that had been rubbed or scratched, and had even raised an imperfect scab, to detain what moisture he could from beneath it to vaccinate with.

If a contagion be so very liable to be changed or modified, in cases of artificial propagation, is it not more likely to become deteriorated in the course of an epidemic, where the subject's exposure, the constitution of him and the patient, the period of the disease at the time of exposure, and the other circumstances, are purely accidental. No contagious disease, as we have before said, is alike infectious *at all stages of its course;* but a difference of a day or two, in this respect, will render the same patient either more or less dangerous to those who approach him. Although, therefore, a disease, resembling the one with which the person is affected at the time, may appear in persons exposed at different periods of his malady, yet it is more than probable that many of them are incomplete and spurious forms only, and, therefore, they are incapable either of affording after-security against a second attack, or sometimes of further propagation at the time of their occurrence.

Unusual determinations to particular organs have been sometimes observed in epidemic diseases. These appear to be purely accidental, and rather the effects of weather, than of any peculiar property in the disease itself. When such symptoms are added (for instance, a violent purging or bowel-complaint), we have no doubt but they exert a powerful influence, even on a genuine contagious malady. By lessening the process of expulsion by the skin, so common in every contagious disease, they may diminish its contagious powers, perhaps destroy them altogether.

We have had no opportunities of learning how far individuals labouring under jaundice, a disease in which the bile is diffused over the whole system, have their susceptibilities to contagion increased or diminished ; or, if jaundiced persons are liable to infection, whether or not the disease in them would prove equally infectious to others.

This part of medicine, the influence of diseases upon one another, has been much neglected, and many circumstances of almost daily occurrence in contagious diseases are still but imperfectly known. Thus, the diagnosis or mode of distinguishing one contagious disease from another is still matter of dispute amongst medical men. Small-pox has been confounded with chicken-pox, scarlet fever with measles, typhus with plague or simple fever, Egyptian or contagious with common ophthalmia, yellow with marsh or bilious fever, and true syphilis with the many diseases that resemble it in appearance, even by physicians of great experience. The different varieties of the same disease have still more frequently been the subject of dispute, and doubts have arisen whether they are of the same species, or totally different diseases. Most writers have described several modifications and anomalous kinds of small-pox. The scientific Willan has divided measles into three species, viz. Rubeola vulgaris, R. sine catarrho, and R. nigra. Spurious kinds of cow-pox were pointed out by Jenner, even on the cow and horse. Three kinds of scarlet fever are described by authors, viz. mitis, anginosa, and maligna; and disputes have arisen whether scarlet fever and malignant sore throat are different diseases, or only varieties of the same disease. The French writers on plague have specified five varieties of that disease; Dr. Russel extended them to six; while Sir Brooke Faulkener and Dr. Pearson restrict them to three. The contentions about syphilis and yellow fever would fill a volume; and a book has been published at Stratsburg to prove that the venereal disease never had existence.—See *the Review of it in Edinburgh Medical Journal*, vol. xiv. *p.* 357.

We have not mentioned these facts as subjects of reproach against the members of a difficult profession, but rather with a view of shewing the great necessity there is for caution in giving opinions. In short, it is impossible to decide on the nature of many diseases, even of common occurrence, by appearances alone; but regard must be paid to the history from beginning to end, not merely of individual cases of the disease, but to the rise, progress, and decline of the epidemic. Diseases specifically contagious have always been, and ever will be, modified by circumstances. To attempt, therefore, to fix certain characters to each, or lay down precise rules for their mode of procedure, is to decide upon the colour of the chameleon, or to fix that which is subject to frequent change.

The different varieties of the same disease, mentioned by authors, are never all alike contagious, nor is the same species alike so at all times of an epidemic, much less in different epidemics. Some varieties, which put on less of the appearance of the true disease, may, nevertheless, be highly contagious; others, having more the appearance, possess no power of propagation: some, again, are not infectious at the first, but become so during their course; while many epidemics, highly contagious at their commencement, begin to decline at a certain stage of their progress, on the principles we have already endeavoured to explain.

These principles are further illustrated by analogy.

Wheat is not a native of Britain, and the seed requires to be renewed, as it degenerates in the course of time on our soil.

Hereditary diseases frequently disappear in families in the course of lineal transmission, or they are latent in one generation and become active in the next.

The healthy secretions are subject to material change from different causes. A young nurse, in a good state of health, has more milk, and milk of a better quality, than one who is old, infirm, or diseased. Whatever disturbs the system of a nurse, when suckling a child, will affect both the quantity and quality of this fluid; and the bad effects of the change it undergoes are soon discoverable upon the child she nurses.

The seminal fluid loses its power of propagation by the presence of a venereal taint in the system of a man. A gentleman, who consulted a physician with whom we are acquainted as to the cause of barrenness in his wife, was advised to undergo a course of mercury, though he was in apparent good health at the time, merely because he had had syphilis some years before. This remedy had the desired effect, his lady becoming pregnant soon after the course was finished.

In 1813, an officer of the navy had his thigh-bone fractured, a little above its lower extremity, in an action with a French frigate. No callus was formed for more than four months after the accident, and, as the patient had no fever, pain, or inflammation, he sometimes amused his sea friends who visited him on shore, by throwing about the broken limb like a flail. At length a venereal taint being suspected in his constitution, although he had not had any symptoms for a length of time, he was put under a course of mercury, and then sent to the country, as we afterwards learnt, with complete success.

We have observed the perspiration to undergo frequent changes in its sensible qualities in a hot climate. Sometimes it is so acid that the sour smell is intolerable. A curious proof of this came to our knowledge. A young lady who was universally admired for her beauty at New South Wales, took a passage on board of one of our merchant ships which touched at the Island of Otaheite on her passage home to Europe. As this lady was probably one of the first English beaut:es that had ever visited this spot, so celebrated for its females, a British officer who happened to be there at the time was anxious to learn the opinion of the natives concerning her. They all allowed this lady to be very handsome and pretty, but said they did not like to be near her, as she had a sour smell. At other times the perspiration is more alkaline, and it bites the eyes and shrivels the skin like the alkali of soap. At a third time it possesses none of these qualities, but is thick, bland, and unctuous.

The urine in diabetes loses its natural qualities, and abounds with saccharine matter. When the Gentoo first discovers that the bees are attracted to a spot by his urine, he knows it is time to make his will.

In an extensive wound, where there is fracture or loss of bone, at first bony matter is deposited, then granulations or growth of flesh takes place, and lastly skin is formed ; yet the least thing affecting the health of the patient will disturb these different sanative processes. An error in diet or treatment, often destroys the progress of a month towards a cure. In like manner, the pus secreted by an abscess, or even the whole ulcers in a large hospital, frequently undergo material changes in the course of a single night.

Thus we see, that the natural secretions are liable to be changed from slight causes. These changes cannot be well accounted for; but, as Nature has taken care to provide particular organs for the regular elaboration of each, we should expect them to be less influenced by adventitious or accidental causes than the morbid secretions. In other words, that the animal system should be more regular and uniform in the performance of a natural function than in one which is unnatural. As the formation of certain morbid poisons is restricted to a few days in a long life, the elaboration of contagion in the human system, would seem to be one of its greatest efforts, and therefore the most unnatural of all, being one which it is never, or at least seldom called upon to repeat. If this view of the subject be correct, is it surprising that the function should often be imperfectly performed, particularly " *in old, weak, and emaciated persons,*" whose systems are incapable of entering into the same degrees of morbid action with those of the " young, healthy, and robust ?" Is it surprising that the contagious principle derived from the body of a diseased person at one stage of the process, should possess a less power over the systems of others than that which is elaborated at another stage ? Is it surprising that the process itself, like every other in the animal economy, should be liable to interruption and change by other morbid or healthy actions incompatible with itself ?

SEASON.—7th. *The last cause of the decline of an epidemic we mentioned is, that the season less favourable to the operation of contagion has now set in.*

Dr. Adams, when speaking of the *true* contagions, observes that, " they may not only be conveyed at any season, climate, or temperature ; but, under all these circumstances, every person affected with either is contagious. It is highly important to mark this difference, because, in those epidemics *which depend on season, climate, or constitution of the atmosphere,* we may look *with certainty* to their termination ; and even hospital fever may be exterminated *by free ventilation. But none of these prevents the spreading of a true contagion."—On Epidemics, p.* 21.

Now, where Dr. Adams found a contagion independent of climate, season, and free ventilation, we cannot even conjecture.

SMALL-POX.—The dependance of small-pox, a true contagion, on season, was remarked by Sydenham : " In the year 1667," says he, " at the approach of the vernal equinox, the small-pox, which, during the immediate preceding pestilential constitution, appeared very rarely, or not at all, began to shew itself, and spreading more and more every day, became epidemic about Autumn ; after which its virulence being abated by degrees, on the coming on of the Winter it decreased, *but returned again the following Spring,* and prevailed till it was checked as before by the subsequent Winter. It afterwards increased a third time *with the approaching Spring,* but did not then rage so severely, nor so generally as it had done the two preceding Summers ; and in August, 1669, it totally disappeared, and was succeeded by an epidemic dysentery."—*P.* 94. The works of this illustrious writer abound with facts, marking the dependance of contagious epidemical diseases on season and atmospheric constitutions. We may likewise remark, that what he here says about small-pox can easily be explained on the principles we have laid down. The disappearance of small-pox during the immediate preceding pestilential constitution ; its appearance when it was ended ; its raging in Summer and ceasing in Winter ; and its total disappearance the third Autumn, when its fuel was expended, accord exactly with what has been said.

The celebrated Boerhave has an aphorism which marks

the same course in small-pox. "This disease," he observes, " is generally epidemical, beginning *early in the Spring, increasing in Summer, abating in Autumn, ceasing almost entirely* the following Winter, to return again in the Spring, and reign again *in the same order*." Van Swieten, the commentator on these aphorisms, remarks—" I have seen many variolous epidemic constitutions, and they agreed in most things with the observations of Sydenham."

Dr. Thomas, in his Modern Practice of Physic, and other practical writers, make similar remarks on small-pox. In the last epidemic at Norwich, an account of which we have given, the small-pox was introduced in the latter part of 1818; but, owing to the cold of Winter, did not begin to spread much till February, 1819, its usual time. "Of the 530 deaths (says Mr. Cross), 298 occurred *in June and July ;* and in June, when the greatest mortality occurred from small-pox, 43 were buried in one week. In like manner (adds he), in the town of Lynn, the small-pox was introduced early in 1819, but did not spread with rapidity until *the warm season*." The knowledge of this general fact, as we are informed by Dr. Monro, led the Bramins of India to begin inoculating for the small-pox in the month of February ; and Mr. C. thinks that, if the people of Norwich could have been made aware of this fact at the time the disease began to spread, and vaccinated, they would have effectually arrested the progress of the epidemic.

We have already stated that the harmattan, a dry wind which blows on the Western Coast of Africa, effectually puts an end to all epidemics, as the small-pox, and that infection, at such a time, does not appear to be easily communicated, even by art.

Cow-Pox.—*Cow-pox, a true Contagion, is also dependant on Season.*

Dr. Woodville, the physician to the Small-pox Hospital, observes—" Unfortunately, at the time Dr. Jenner's publication appeared, no cow-pox matter could be procured, for the disease *had then become extinct;* nor was it expected to return till *the Spring,* the period at which it *usually* affects the cows. Towards the latter end of January last, I was informed that the cow-pox had appeared on several of the milch-cows kept in Gray's-Inn Lane, and about four-fifths of them were eventually infected."

In Germany, the cow-pox is apparently so extinct at one time, and so prevalent at another, that it is the belief of some scientific men that *it is newly originated.* According to Pilger, a veterinary surgeon, the disease arises among the cattle in Russia when they are driven to Moscow.*

MEASLES.—Of measles, another true contagion, Sydenham says :—" In the beginning of January, 1671, the measles appeared, *as is usual,* and increased daily till the approach of the vernal equinox, when it came to its height, after which it abated in the same gradual manner, and went quite off in July following."—*P.* 161.

SCARLATINA.—The same author observes, that "the scarlet fever may happen at any time, yet it generally comes at *the close of Summer,* when it seizes whole families, but especially children." This disease has become much more formidable since his time; in proof of which Sydenham remarks —" As the disease seems to me to be nothing more than a *moderate efflorescence* of the blood, occasioned by *the heat of the preceding Summer,* or some other way, I do nothing that may prevent the desquamation of the blood, and the expulsion of the peccant matter through the pores, which *is quickly enough performed.*"—*P.* 226. At the present day, we have seen no contagious disease sometimes so quickly proving fatal in Britain as scarlet fever.

---

* See some excellent observations, in the 33d volume of the Quarterly Review.

HOOPING-COUGH.—Hooping-cough, the last true contagion, in the sense some consider the term, although it is put
down as the least contagious of all others in the scale of the
learned Dr. Parr, seems to be every way as dependant on
season as those we have mentioned. Every experienced physician knows that it generally prevails in *cold damp seasons*,
as the end of *Autumn* and *Winter*, and is little heard of in
the warm dry days of Summer.

It is not necessary to enlarge the evidence on this head ;
what has been stated being sufficient to shew, that the influence of season and atmospheric constitutions on the true
contagions had not only been long remarked, but that this dependance appeared to be so conspicuous to the older authors,
as to mislead them into a belief that certain peculiarities, or
manifest changes, of air were the only agents in operation.
The same error still prevails with regard to some other contagions. We shall not insult the good sense of our readers
by questioning, for a moment, the contagious nature of plague
and typhus fever. Dr. Bancroft, who may be accounted a
high authority on this point, having written a masterly essay
to prove that yellow fever is not contagious, candidly admits
the contagion of both.

YELLOW FEVER.—" The constant extinction of yellow fever by frost (says Dr. B.), is one of those points in which it
resembles the marsh, and *only* the marsh fever. This in-
structive and highly important fact is, however, capable of
more extensive application ; for it not only proves the origin
and nature of all these fevers, but it also proves decidedly
that the yellow fever has no power of propagating itself by
contagion, *consequently, that it never proceeds from it.*"—
Essay, p. 425. Yet the very same author, when speaking of
plague, which he considers a *highly contagious disease*, says:

PLAGUE.—" The cold in Egypt is never sufficient to stop
the progress of plague ; but in Russia, Poland, and *even in*

Great Britain, the Winter has commonly produced *an almost total cessation of it."—Essay, p.* 592. And, at p. 605, he notices the fact of its being rendered nearly, if not completely, extinct in Britain by the cold of Winter. We would ask—how, then, does it happen that the extinction of yellow fever by frost proves decidedly *that it is never contagious ?* If, in this point of extinction by frost, it resembles the marsh, and *only* the marsh fever, and is, therefore, not contagious, why does it so closely resemble plague, a highly contagious disease, that the one is extinguished by frost, the other almost totally extinguished by even the cold of Winter in Great Britain ? Is the cold of Winter at New York, which extinguishes yellow fever, less on the *Continent* of North America than the cold of Winter in the *Island* of Great Britain, which is commonly sufficient to produce an almost total cessation of plague ? If the Winter, in the Island of Britain, be sufficient to check the operation of *the gross and palpable* matter of plague and small-pox, is it wonderful that the Winters on the Continents of Europe and America should be capable of arresting the propagating power of *the subtle and impalpable gaseous contagion of yellow fever ?*

" Dr. Mertins tells us (continues Dr. Bancroft) that, after the month of October (in the great plague of Moscow), there was a great diminution in the number of attacks and of their mortality ; and this is more accurately proved by the statements given by Orræus, at p. 48, by which it appears that the deaths, in September, were 21,404 ; in October, 17,561 ; in November, 5,235 ; in December, 805; in January, 320."— *Bancroft, p.* 593. " People *newly* employed (Dr. B. adds) in the service of the sick, as barbers, nurses, &c. though still exposed in attending patients at the hospital, scarcely any of them had it *after the month of November,* and these *only in a mild form."—Ibid.* But we have more proof to offer of the dependance of the great plague of Moscow on season.

The first patient died in the military hospital so early as November, 1770, the year before it raged ; but it was not till the 23d of December following, by which time about a *dozen* of persons had died in the neighbourhood of the hospital, that the physicians pronounced the disease to be plague. The hospital was then placed in quarantine, and all the persons who had been seized were also separated, and their clothes and furniture burnt. The weather became intensely cold, *and, all traces of the contagion being lost,* the people passed from a cautious fear to a fearless security. The communication with the hospital was opened in February; but, on the 11th of March, the physicians were again convoked, in consequence of the disease again appearing. After this, *it increased gradually as the season advanced,* till it proved fatal to upwards of 80,000 *persons in Moscow alone.* The disease began to decline in October, as we have seen, and at length finally ceased with the year. Had this plague been introduced into Moscow at a more favourable season, the progress of the epidemic at the beginning must have been more rapid.

" These facts (says Dr. Bancroft, after the words we last quoted from him) will enable us, in a great degree, to understand why, notwithstanding the contagious nature of plague, an exposure to its contagion is frequently harmless; and it is fortunate for mankind that Divine Providence has made its communication to depend upon the co-operation of so many favourable circumstances, *and particularly that of a suitable temperature,* that of its application by actual contact, probably continued for some time, and that of certain aptitude and susceptibility in the human subject; for without such requisites, or such obstacles to the propagation of the disease, the earth might have long since become desolate."—*P.* 593.

In these sentiments concerning plague every one must agree with Dr. B.; but, as that gentleman observes of the extinction of yellow fever by frost, " they admit of more extensive application;" for the close resemblance of yellow fever, in these respects, to plague and other contagious diseases, and, on the other hand, its dissimilarity, in many essential points to be afterwards noticed, to marsh fever, decidedly prove it to be of the same class, consequently, that it is a contagious disease, though, like them, not capable of propagation in every season, and under all circumstances alike.*

A great number of facts might be adduced as further proof of this resemblance.

In the great plague of 1665, " There died (says the historian) more that week, viz. from the 25th July to the 1st August, in the two parishes of Cripplegate and St. Sepulchre, by forty-eight, than in all the city, all the west suburbs, and all the Southwark parishes put together."—*P.* 383. This was the season most favourable to the contagion of plague and the two parishes specified, happened to be places where it then raged.

The yellow fever of Cadiz, in 1800, was introduced at a season favourable to its operation ; like the plague of West Barbary, its progress was unusually rapid, as, in both places, besides season being favourable to their spreading, the constitutions of the people in both instances were unprotected by any previous attack. The number of persons attacked with the fever of Cadiz, according to Sir James Fellowes, from the beginning of August to the first week in November,

* Dr. Bancroft, speaking of the effect of heat in lessening the susceptibilities of individuals to plague, says, at p. 590, " it was most evident in persons who had lately arrived from cold climates ;" and he ascribes his own escape to this, and adds, " there were, however, persons in Egypt who had been long accustomed to greater degrees of heat, and who were, therefore, not rendered insusceptible of plague, and some few of these caught it, *after it had become extinct in the British army,* and when a person recently landed from England would not receive it, *though he slept in an infected bed ;* and it was from this cause that, in the Autumn of the same year, the disease began at Rosetta, two months nearly before the usual time, in natives of the East Indies, and it was propagated with some rapidity, for six or eight weeks, among persons who were either born in, or had just come from a climate much hotter than Egypt, whilst the British troops directly from England did not receive, and probably could not have been made to take the disease." We have quoted the above passage merely to show the faith of the author in the power of temperature on a true contagion.

1800, amounted to 48,688 (*p.* 50,) out of a population reckoned at 57,499 (*Appendix,*) it therefore results that 8,979 escaped.

At Gibraltar, in 1804, when the yellow fever appeared for the first time, only twenty-eight persons escaped an attack out of 14,000, the civil population; and 5,946 persons, including military, died from the 28th August, at which time it began, and all disease ceased by the 1st of January, 1805. Twelve hundred soldiers, out of a garrison containing 4,200, were saved by proper measures of precaution.

The population of Seville, in 1800, and before yellow fever appeared there, according to the official statement, amounted to 80,968. Of these 76,488 were attacked with the prevailing fever, 4,480 escaped, 61,718 recovered, 14,685 died. The yellow fever appeared in Seville about the 23d of August. The following is a list of the number of deaths in each month : Nine days of August 165, September 2106, October 9236, November 1223.—*Sir James Fellowes' Reports, p.* 421.

Yellow fever never appears in North America, or in the South of Europe, but in that season when the heat favours its spreading. We have already seen that the cold of Moscow nearly suppressed the plague of 1770-1, and that the Winter checked almost entirely the epidemic small-pox in Norwich, in the years 1818-19, and that of 530 deaths, 298 happened in June and July of the latter year. Why then should the dependance of yellow fever on season be marked out as a peculiarity.

In warmer climates, plague is much influenced by weather. South wind, says Baron Larrey, increases, North wind diminishes plague in Egypt. Plague, adds he, is contagious and epidemic, not when *slight* or in its *first* stage, not by feeling the pulse, not from dressing buboes, not touching a small surface of the body or clothes of whatever kind they be, or from going into the sick room if there be *a current of air.* Few cases of the yellow fever at Gibraltar proved fatal in

December; and, as soon as the weather became moderately cool, the convalescents recovered rapidly.—*Pym.*

M. Volney observes, " L'Hiver detruit la peste à Constantinople, parceque la froid y est très rigoureux; l'Eté l'allume, parceque la chaleur y est humides, à raison des mers, des forêts, et des montagnes voisines. En Egypt, l'Hiver fomente la peste, parcequ'il est humide et doux; l'Eté la detruit, parcequ'il est chaud et sec."

The influence of a high temperature, in putting a stop to the progress of plague, is very well known. In Egypt, Syria, and Turkey—in the whole of the Levant and coast of Barbary, the people look to St. John's day, or the 24th of June, as a certain period for its termination. Then the heat is much increased, and *heavy dews* resembling rain begin to fall. We do not offer proof of a fact so well known and so generally acknowledged. Doctor Bancroft is of opinion, that plague cannot propagate either in a *hot* or very *cold* climate ; and, on the other hand, that typhus fever is confined to a *cold* or *temperate* region. Most of our best writers coincide in this opinion.

The minor contagions are likewise influenced by climate. We have seen every symptom, primary and secondary, of the venereal disease, disappear without medicine, by removal to a warm latitude, remain latent in the system while the patient continued there, yet return when he arrived in Britain, and being finally removed by a long course of mercury. Sir Gilbert Blane, found that ship's crews affected with itch on leaving England, got better of it without any remedy on arriving in warmer latitudes. The Egyptian or contagious ophthalmia, was much milder in Britain than in Egypt. On the other hand, hydrophobia, which appears often in Britain, is never, according to Baron Larrey, seen in Egypt. Although a true contagion, like all those diseases we have mentioned, yet with us it is confined chiefly to a certain season, so well known that they have been called the dog days. No one has

ever claimed this as a marsh disease. Like every other contagion, it prevails more in some seasons or years than in
others. Mr. Abernethy saw eighty-two cases of it during
his apprenticeship in the London Hospital, but no case
occurred for several years afterwards. In countries, however, possessing a more uniform high temperature, such as
India, Malta, and Egypt, the disease is either seldom seen or
altogether unknown.

Having now adduced sufficient proof of the influence of
climate and season, on all contagious diseases, viz. small
and cow-pox, measles, scarlet fever, hooping-cough, plague,
yellow and typhus fever, venereal disease, itch, ophthalmia,
and hydrophobia, and explained, to the best of our understanding, the different phenomena connected with the rise,
progress, decline, and final termination of a contagious epidemic, we shall finish this part of our subject with a few
general observations. We consider these necessary, notwithstanding the length to which we have already gone, as
perhaps no subject connected with the history of disease, has
given rise to so much error, or to errors of the same pernicious tendency. Any one who will take the trouble of
attentively considering the principles laid down, all of which
we have supported by facts, must be convinced of the utter
impossibility of explaining all the phenomena connected
with epidemics on any single principle. He who looks
for an explanation to the atmosphere, will find, it is true,
that certain contagions are much confined to certain climates :
that plague prevails in Egypt Turkey, Syria, and the
Levant; typhus fever in Britain; yellow fever in the West
Indies; yaws in a few parts of Scotland; plica in Poland, &c.
but he will likewise find a number of other countries which,
although they be placed in the same latitudes, and possess
similar climates and seasons, are nevertheless exempted
from any such distempers. He will observe, in the same
country, seasons exactly similar in point of heat, dryness,
moisture, and prevailing winds, yet have quite oppo-

site effects on the public health—that the appearance of
epidemics, therefore, does not depend upon season alone—
that their progress and duration in a place, are influenced
by the time they have been absent from it—that the same
contagion never prevails to a great extent for two succeeding
years—that, when it prevails to a smaller extent the first
year, it may re-appear in the succeeding ; or, like the epidemic
small-pox mentioned by Sydenham, even in a third—that
the beginning of epidemics is frequently accidental, and that
their end or duration depends upon their beginning, or on the
rapidity of their course—that when they appear early in the
year, and spread rapidly throughout, they will terminate in
that season which is supposed to be most favourable : on
the contrary, that, when they appear late, they will continue
to rage beyond their usual time, finally,—that, when they
are regular in their time of appearing, they will be more
regular in their course and final cessation.

He must be convinced upon reflection, that the usual mode
of calculating the power of season on epidemic diseases is extremely fallacious. The fact of one hundred persons being
attacked with a disease in the month of April, and ten thousand
in the month of August, cannot be received as proof that the
latter season is one hundred times more favourable to the
contagion than the former one ; but he must recollect that
ten sick persons will produce ten times more contagion than
one ; one hundred, ten times more than ten ; a thousand, ten
times more than a hundred, and so on ; till the supply of
subjects susceptible to its influence becomes exhausted.

We have, therefore, in reality, no proof that the great heat
of the month of August is one whit more favourable to the
disease, than the lower temperature of the month of April.

If, after raging for some months, a disease ceases suddenly
in the month of November, this cannot be received as any
evidence of the power of cold and frost in checking its progress. As plague and yellow fever frequently perform as
much work in six weeks as some other diseases do in six

months, they must sooner exhaust that supply of subjects on which alone they depend, or at least without which they cannot exist.

If, however, a disease which is first introduced into a city in the latter end of the year languish, or remain dormant during the cold season, and be resuscitated by warmer weather, as happened in the plague of Moscow and the small-pox of the towns of Norwich and Lynn as before mentioned, this without doubt is a fair demonstration of the influence of season on a contagious malady.* If a single person labouring under a contagious disease prove uniformly more dangerous to all having communication with him in the month of August, than an individual under the same circumstances in the month of April, this too must be admitted as legitimate evidence of the power of season. But whether the increase of temperature, in the latter instance, adds activity to the contagion formed, or merely enables the system of the sick person to secrete a greater quantity of the poison, is quite a different question, and one which cannot be so easily solved.

The instances adduced of the influence of the atmosphere, do not warrant us to conclude that epidemics do occur independent of a definite and specific agent, or that the cause arises from any peculiar state of air in regard to its physical or chemical qualities. The agency of these properties are known to be the same in every part of the globe and at every known height from the earth's surface ; and any alterations they occasionally undergo, have been ascertained to be partial only, so that their effects can never be felt beyond the sphere of their action.

No quality of the atmosphere, physical, chemical, electrical or other, could possibly afford an explanation of the slow and gradual progress of an epidemic at its beginning,

---

* In giving the proof of the influence of season on the plague of Moscow, Dr. Bancroft has quoted from Orræus the fallacious facts of its greater mortality in September, and its decline after this period. Where had the disease more susceptible subjects ?

nor of its after-spreading in every direction, often contrary to
the wind, being alike independent of the heavenly bodies, the
laws of gravity, those which regulate caloric and the electric
fluid, and regardless of the chemical properties of that
heterogeneous mass of matter constituting the organic structure of the earth. To believe in such an agent, is to believe
in the existence of a thing arising from nothing, yet being independent of every thing. Where contagion is genuine, and
the circumstances of society are favourable to an epidemic,
the usual effects of season will not be observed.

The second plague of Athens, according to Thucydides,
broke out in the beginning of Winter, yet it proved fatal in a
very short time to 4,000 foot soldiers, and 300 cavalry, with
a proportional number of inhabitants. Galen likewise mentions a plague having invaded Aquileia in the middle of Winter.
The plague of Constantinople has proved fatal to 1,000 persons a day, at a time when the streets were covered with
snow. It raged at Malta in 1813, when the thermometer
was between 80 and 90 degrees. Muratori relates that " la
peste dell 1630, fu al somno a Padova ne mesi de Giugno et
Luglio, *ma in Venezia la stessa fore strages maggiore nell
Ottobre, Novembre et Decembre, continuando per tutte
l'anno sequente,* 1631, sempre diminenda " Sydenham,
Dover, Mead, and others give many similar instances of
pestilential diseases appearing during Winter and remaining
through that and the succeeding seasons. St. John's day
does not always put a stop to epidemic plague. In the yellow
fever of Philadelphia in 1793, several deaths happened in
December : Sir James Fellowes has given a table of twenty-
three towns where it appeared in Spain in 1804. In Vera
it was most fatal on *the 30th day of November,* and it did
not cease till the 4th of January, 1805. In Guardana, the
most fatal day was the 12*th of November,* and it ceased
on the 16th. In Arcos, the 25*th of November* was the most
fatal, and the place was declared healthy on the 3d of
December. In Villa Martin, the disease was at its height by

the 15th of November; declared healthy 25th December. In Ximenes de la Frontera, the 30th November was the most fatal, and it was declared healthy exactly a month afterwards. Carthagena de Levante, where 11,445 persons died, was not declared healthy till the 23d of January, 1805. There was only one town out of all the twenty-three which the table contains, which was declared free from the disease before the month of November.

The season at Gibraltar in 1813, when the yellow fever raged, was one of the healthiest, in other respects, in remembrance; and it is well known that fresh subjects were attacked on coming to Cadiz, and other parts of Spain, after the yellow fever had ceased in those places.

It may be contended, it is true, that a disease may continue in individuals labouring under it for some time after its cause has ceased to operate on persons in health—that, therefore, the period of its ceasing in a place is no criterion for judging of the exact time when the morbid agent was destroyed by season. But this argument would have double force against marsh fevers, which are known to be diseases of a long and indefinite course, to what it would have against yellow fever, a disease in most instances of only a few days' duration.

If yellow fever be constantly destroyed by frost, it must be unlike marsh fevers, which would continue, agreeable to this argument, long after the cold has set in; for, according to Dr. Bancroft, marsh poison may remain latent in the system for months, or for almost any intermediate period between that and a few days. If this opinion of his be correct, how does it happen that frost, as he says also, constantly extinguishes marsh fever; or, who could say when, or by what marsh poison is destroyed. The atmospheric philosopher will, moreover, find that, before the year 1720, the city of Marseilles had no plague for seventy years; before 1813, Malta had escaped for 138 years; before 1770, Moscow was free for 150 years; and that the great fire of London in 1666, banished it from the bills of mortality of that city—that plague has not always infested Egypt or Turkey; that places like the citadel of Cairo and the village in West Barbary, though in the immediate neighbourhood of terrible epidemics, remained healthy; and, lastly, that this frightful malady has never yet reached any part of the New World, although it possesses every climate and every season favourable to its existence. Similar facts will be mentioned in the history of yellow fever.

With respect to the small-pox, measles, scarlet fever, and hooping-cough, he will find New Holland still exempted from their ravages, although this large island (like America for plague,) possesses every climate and season known to be favourable to their presence. Their progress in other parts of the globe, in most instances, can be distinctly traced to have arisen from intercourse and communication between one portion of it and another. Accordingly, from those parts of Asia which were first peopled they gradually spread over the rest of the world, and their first appearance in some quarters of it is generally acknowledged to be within the limits of well authenticated history. The mode of spreading observable in all the diseases we have mentioned, is, therefore, one of those points in their history that cannot be mistaken. If there were no other, this alone is sufficient to stamp their character, and to demonstrate their dependance on some cause unconnected with the atmosphere.

As Doctor Robertson has well observed, it is impossible to comprehend how a change in the physical properties of the atmosphere, capable of engendering any general disease, should take place without other circumstances connected with that change upon other bodies becoming manifest. If such happened, every one should be affected at *nearly the same time*, as, in every condition of the atmosphere, it must act upon man and all respiring animals in nearly a similar manner. What then shall we say of the diseases above-

* Natural History of the Atmosphere, Vol. ii. p. 321.

mentioned. All of them have been observed to rage sometimes in one town and not in the next; in one street and
not in the adjoining one; in one side of a street before it
appears on the opposite; in one house and not in another;
in one room of a house and not in the adjoining apartment of
the same dwelling. None of them affect a whole community
at nearly the same time; they spread not generally, but from
individual to individual; they appear in seasons where no
change in the physical or chemical properties are manifested,
either by philosophical experiments, by common observation,
or by any evident corresponding changes on respiring animals
in general, or on the vegetable kingdom; and we know that
seasons exactly similar produce none of those diseases. What
then becomes of the mere atmospheric dogmatic, driven
by all the above facts from point to point, and from something to nothing? his only resource must be to take shelter
under his inexplicables and incomprehensibles, in order to
excuse his ignorance.

The mere contagionist or the believer in the omnipotence
of the agent, contagion, itself, must likewise find himself frequently in error. He cannot agree with Dr. Adams, in believing the true contagions to be independent of climate,
season, and atmospheric constitutions, if he read the proofs
of such dependance, which have been given by almost all
the best writers, ancient and modern. Still it must appear
evident to him, that the atmosphere is oftentimes an *ac-
cessary*, but never an *essential* cause of epidemic contagious
diseases.

Lastly, he who looks for an explanation to the condition of
society *alone*, will not *at first* be more fortunate than the
atmospheric and contagionist; for he will find that filth, vice,
famine, misery, and wretchedness, do not *always* generate
contagion. Upon more mature reflection, however, he will
come nearer his mark. He will become convinced, that nothing but the body of a living animal can produce contagion,
but that things external, may induce or excite the diseased

action in the animal system by which it may be generated.
In short, that the contagions have, in all ages in which they
were known, maintained a close and intimate connexion exclusively with the animal system, which is not always merely
acted upon by a cause arising from things unconnected with
itself, but by one which it alone has the power of forming.
In other words, the contagions are animal secretions.

This first step being gained, his next inquiry will be, what
condition of a living animal is required to form a contagion ?
A state of disease is the only answer that can be given to
this question; consequently, the contagions are not healthy,
but morbid animal secretions. The third question which he
wishes to have solved is, what species of animal is capable
of forming those secretions during disease ? Hydrophobia
arises from the canine species ; vaccine matter from the cow
and horse ; all the other contagions are probably confined to
the human species. To his fourth question, are all the human
species equally liable to fall into that diseased condition
which is required to form contagion ? the answer is sufficiently
manifest. In proportion as man deviates from certain laws
pointed out by nature, in the same proportion will he become
liable to disease.

The wandering savage, if he only wash the surface of his
naked body, may derive contagion from others, but he is not
so likely to fall into that diseased condition which produces
it. Whatever may be his hunger or his toils, still he will be
free. Without habitation to deprive him of a constant
supply of fresh air, without clothing to accumulate human
effluvia, he is exempted in his natural state from this numerous tribe of maladies, so fatal to other classes of society.
The hunter, fisherman, shepherd, and cultivator of the soil,
possessing settled abodes, and wearing clothes, will run
greater risk than him. The third class, or those who not only
possess settled habitations and wear clothing, but live in
closer society, will be still more exposed ; while those living
in the dirty narrow streets of large towns, will be the fourth

class. The poor of large cities, who can neither afford to have habitations sufficiently large or well ventilated, nor clothing sufficiently clean, will be the fifth ; and the vicious and criminal, who are confined in small cells in a jail, crowded with inmates, as they are deprived of almost every means preventing the accumulation of human effluvia, must be the most exposed of all.

If our knowledge of the subject be allowed to be thus far correct, it cannot fail to be useful. The medical enquirer, it is true, will not be able to tell exactly what combination of mischievous powers is required to generate a contagion ; but, so far as prevention is concerned, his information must prove of much value. He will observe, that the condition of human society most favorable to the generation of contagion is, also, that in which it is afterwards best maintained or kept up.

Generation of Contagion.

Having now examined the different phenomena that have been mentioned by authors, as being connected with the rise, progress, and decline of contagious epidemic diseases, and explained them to the best of our ability on known principles, as laid down in the part on contagion itself, we shall next proceed to notice some other things concerning the morbid poisons, which could not be so conveniently brought in at another part of the work—or at least considered with that attention which their importance seemed to require.

The mode in which a contagion is generated, is one of these. As before hinted, some writers dignify the contagions with many of the attributes of animals, and grant them distinctions superior to vegetables. They divide them into distinct species, though not into different sexes. They give to the disease occasioned by each, distinct forms and characters, which they imagine are always the same, or nearly the same. They deny that the contagions are ever in any case the creatures of circumstances, and they point to direct propagation as the only means by which they can be produced, and by which alone they are preserved from generation to generation in all their original power and purity. So far are they, however, from being independent of circumstances, that we know of few contagious diseases that have not undergone some material change in their nature within the period of well authenticated history. Their characteristic marks are, therefore, far from being well established. Thus, although syphilis has been known in Europe for about 350 years, few surgeons of the present day would trust to their knowledge of its symptoms alone. The Proteian forms of plague, typhus, and yellow fever, are just as proverbial, and the contentions about small-pox and chicken-pox are not yet settled. Upon the whole, although we do not think the animal œconomy so pliable as the vegetable, where the power of art, in varying the appearance, and even the nature of plants, is so conspicuous, still we cannot agree with those authors who give to the contagions inherent qualities and outward characters, every way as distinct and fixed as if they were the animals themselves, instead of being the products only.

Dr. Bancroft finds fault with Dr. Chisholm, for making the contagion, which broke out in the ship Hankey, at Bulama, an equivocal production, without parent or generative agent. " He left it," he says, " as St. Paul describes Melchizedec to have been, without father, without mother, and without descent." But neither Dr. B. nor any other author, has been able to give us a distinct notion of the birth, parentage, or pedigree of any of these morbid poisons. To compare their generation with that of animals is absurd. The matter of contagion is produced by inserting a small quantity of a similar kind, into the body of a healthy animal of *either sex, and of different ages.* Animal propagation requires a certain principle to be derived from the male and female, and a particular function to be performed by each at the same time. In one case it matters not *in what part of the body* the foreign

principle is introduced; in the other, the mode of conveyance is essential. By the introduction of contagion, an
evident change is produced *over the whole system*, and the
mass of fluids is altered; in the other, the change which
follows is more local. The one is attended with *a morbid action* of the system, without which, no new matter is
formed; the other is attended with a comparatively healthy
action. The same contagion cannot be generated in the
same system more than once during life. Animal generation
is likewise restricted within a certain age. It would appear,
therefore, that in the generation of contagion, this new and
morbid action of the animal system, is the creative power;
for the matter has no force or effect in increasing itself without it. Hence, those diseases which pre-occupy the whole
system, and, by so doing, prevent this necessary action, all
confer immunity on the persons so affected from contagion,
even where inoculation has been employed. If the mere in-
sertion of a small quantity of matter had the power of accumulation in the body of animals, *without the constitutional
action*, we see no reason why the generation of contagion
should be restricted in so many instances to once during the
life of any individual. May it not be inferred that the human
body contains within itself all the principles necessary to
form morbid secretions as well as healthy ones? If so, why
may not the contagions be generated therein, without the aid
of matters similar to themselves? The rareness of their production militates against this opinion. But if we consider
the strong incentives Nature has implanted in all animals to
propagate their species, and, on the other hand, the feelings
of horror and disgust, equally strong, which most of them
possess against whatever is offensive to their senses or likely
to injure their health, we shall not wonder if animal generation be the most common occurrence of the two. Besides,
as before said, there is no particular organ of the body set
apart for the purpose of secreting these poisons during health,
as in the case of the viper and some other venomous animals;

but the same organ which is employed for other purposes during health, assumes to itself a new creative power during disease.

This is not the only instance where the animal body changes, or takes on new functions according to circumstances. The mass of blood contains bony matter, which, however, is not deposited in quantity, unless a loss of bone has been sustained in some part or other. *Then, without the aid of any unusual adventitious matters being applied,* the body takes on a whole series of new formative processes. Bone is first generated till the loss be supplied; then soft parts, in rotation, as they are wanted; and lastly, skin. The cyst of an abscess secretes pus till it be destroyed; a raw surface will do the same. The secretion of milk in the breast of the female, takes place only at certain times, and only under certain circumstances; yet *we do not know of any foreign or adventitious agent* which requires to be added to her system, before this secretion begins; neither do we know of any principle being lost during its secretion : for the mass of fluids are the same, so far as we have yet learnt, after the process is finished, as it was before it had begun. That no adventitious agent is added during gestation, which has the property of exciting the lacteal secretion, is evident from the fact that it takes place in the female without sexual intercourse or conception; and milk sometimes appears even in the male breast at different ages, and in that of an infant of either sex. The rudiments of the teeth are contained in the gums of the infant at birth; yet they do not appear till it attains a certain age : and, after two sets of teeth come forward, it is rare, where the body has the power of producing a third.

From all this, then, we have proof of the dependance of the healthy secretions on circumstances. We have no proof *of any extraordinary adventitious agents being necessary* to excite them, far less of any principle being lost during secretion. *It is the function, not the principle which is lost.* It must be confessed, however, that the morbid secretions possess one quality which is peculiar to them ; that is, the power of exciting that morbid action in a healthy system, by which matters similar to themselves are produced. Wherever the morbid action is general and violent, the power of exciting the same is lost. Where contagion acts locally and not violently on the whole system, the generative process may be repeated in the same person any number of times. Some of the healthy secretions are restricted like the morbid ones to a certain age, or to a given number of times during the life of the individual. The power of procreation, menstruation, and the secretion of milk in the female, as also dentition in both sexes are of this kind.

If our view of this mysterious subject be correct, the animal system, as it relates to contagion, may be compared to an egg fitted for incubation. It only requires what may be compared to the heat of the hen or of the oven, namely, certain febrile action, *or excitement* of *the whole system,* continued for a given length of time, to generate it; not always matter similar to itself.

We have a further illustration of this from the fact, that fevers sometimes arising from common causes, and which are not contagious at their beginning, yet become so in the course of their progress without contagious matter of any kind having been applied. Sir J. Pringle, Sir James M'Grigor, Lind, Blane, Burnett, Johnson, Hunter, and Jackson, all medical writers, belonging, or who did belong to the army or navy, as also Cullen, Heberden, Haygarth, Willan, Perceval, Currie, Clark, Good, and a host of other writers, acknowledge this as a fact. Some, indeed, have attempted to draw a distinction between the fevers of this kind, and the specific contagions. Dr. Rush was one who made this distinction. He says, " *that vitiated product of living vascular action,* which can excite in a well person a disease like that by which itself was produced, and continue indefinitely to do so after being transferred from one body to another, will be denominated *contagion;"* and lues, cow-pox, measles, and small-pox, he gives as examples of it. " On the other hand," he adds, " *that venomous offspring of putrefaction,* going on in some of the kinds of organic matter *after death, or separation from the living frame,* which disorders the healthy functions without being specifically communicable, and without the power of communicating itself, will be called *infection ;* and typhus, dysentery, plague, and yellow fever, will be given as instances."—*American Med. Rep.,* vol. vi.

How Dr. Rush could find out that the exhalations arising from a pestilential bubo were less the product of vascular action than those emanating from a venereal bubo, or how he could distinguish that the effluvium arising from a human body under typhus fever was an excretion, and that separated from one in scarlet fever, a secretion, it is impossible to tell ; nor is it now necessary to enquire ; seeing that this distinction has never been shown to be a difference by any of our best writers. The septic theory of Rush* has had few believers. If contagion be produced in this way, in some instances, the comparison between its generation, and the generation and propagation of animals cannot stand. Caloric exists in a latent state in all bodies, and it does not become active, but under certain circumstances. A small spark of fire is generally necessary to ignite an inflammable substance, but we know that many of them are capable of spontaneous combustion. So does the matter seem to stand with contagion. The human system contains within itself all the matters necessary to form contagion, which, however, do not become active, but under certain circumstances. In general,

---

* The fancy of this great man, which was always exuberant, became mystified in his latter days. When he became sceptical as to contagion in yellow fever, he naturally turned septical at the same time. It is a pity that the acidity which characterised the chemical theorists who flourished in the medical repository of those days, did not counteract or neutralize this septic tendency.

a small quantity of contagious matter of the same kind is necessary to excite them into action ; still we know that contagion has been formed spontaneously in the human system. We grant this mode of the generation of contagion to be a very rare occurrence, but so is the spontaneous combustion of the human body ; and perhaps the whole history of human pathology cannot furnish a more remarkable proof of the changes which sometimes take place in the system ; for that body which burns with difficulty when thrown into a fire in *a healthy state,* nevertheless ignites and consumes spontaneously *during disease.*

Unless the poisons generated in plague, typhus, and yellow fever were morbid secretions, the same as other contagions, it seems impossible to conceive how a person visiting another labouring under those diseases should contract, *in all instances,* the same malady with the person he visits. " If he derives any thing specific," says Professor Hossack, " from the sick, his disease is then assuredly to be considered as depending on the peculiar condition of the fluids, or state of the system, induced by the action of a specific poison. In other words, it is to be considered as a contagious disease."—*Letter to Dr. Chisholm.* But by what combination of pestiferous powers, or by what peculiar disposition in our bodies an animal poison is at first generated, is another and a more difficult question. Though dead animal matters, and other kinds of filth, are not in themselves sufficient to produce a contagion, yet it seems certain they sometimes cause fevers which afterwards become contagious. Such matters, therefore, are not merely the entertainers of contagion, but finally become the indirect producers, by enabling the system to form it. A contagion cannot be produced by synthisis without the body, and that putrid animal matters, and other kinds of filth, are often harmless, has been shewn by Dr. Bancroft, and other authors of eminence. It seems not to be the sudden application of such matters for *a short time* that proves injurious in this way; for when such matters, so applied, do prove hurtful to human health, it is by their mephitic quality, or by the exclusion of oxygen or vital air merely, of course, death ensues, *before the accession of the necessary febrile action.* To suppose that a contagion might be formed under such circumstances, is to look for an effect without a cause; for, according to the vulgar Scotch proverb, it is like " *killing* the cow and expecting the milk."*

It is the application of human effluvia, and other kinds of filth *for a length of time, keeping the body in a state of disease, or one analagous to disease,* that is most likely to generate contagion.

* " In the month of September, 1784, a poor woman died in the hospital at Aberdeen, and was buried in a church-yard in the neighbourhood. A company of young surgeons agreed with the grave-digger to set a mark on the grave, as a direction for them to find the body for anatomical purposes; but some person, in order to disappoint the grave-digger's employers, moved the signal to another grave, that of a woman who had been buried three or four months. The party came, and, directed by the mark agreed on, dug up the grave, drew out the coffin and carried it home. But upon opening it, a vapour like fume of brimstone came forth, and suffocated them in an instant. Two women also going past the room fell down dead, and it was said that eleven persons perished from the baneful effluvia."—*Taylor on Premature Interment, P.* 115. No contagion could be formed here. But where the persons exposed to such vapours survive long enough to pass through fever, the case is very different. Cotte, in his Treatise on Meteorology, gives a case of this kind, which happened at Montmorency, in 1773. A vapour arose from the coffin of a person recently buried, during the time of a funeral, and out of 120 persons present, 114 took ill of a putrid and *venomous* fever. A school-boy at West Linton, some years ago, getting into a new made grave, set about to open the projecting corner of a coffin, which as soon as he had penetrated, there issued from thence a strong noxious smell, on which he exclaimed he was suffocated; he revived on being taken out of the place, but fell immediately ill of a pestilential fever, of which he died on the seventh day. By this means a similar fever was communicated to some of the people who had attended him during his illness.— *See Dr. Robertson on the Natural History of the Atmosphere.*

The following circumstances have been blamed by some of our best writers, as being those most likely to generate contagious fevers :—

1st. Effluvia arising from the bodies of people in health, when shut up in narrow confined places.

2nd. Effluvia of sick people under similar circumstances.

3rd. Effluvia from putrid bodies.

4th. Unusual condition of the air, and especially sudden and violent changes of weather, to which the system cannot always adapt itself.

5th. Filth, intemperance, insolations, fatigue, want, excess of venery, passions of the mind, or any debilitating cause.

Dr. Lind, mentions an instance of a frigate, on its passage from North America to England, on board of which, he says, "a seasoned sound crew became infected, as it would appear, from the closeness or dampness below, occasioned by the hatchways being shut up."—*On Fevers and Infection,* cap. i., 32.

Sir John Pringle, has observed, in his work on the Diseases of the Army, that contagious fever is incidental to every place ill aired and kept dirty, that is filled with animal steams from foul and diseased bodies; and, therefore, that the hospitals of an army, not only when crowded with sick, but at any time when the air is confined, but especially in hot weather, produce a fever of a pestilential kind. He makes similar remarks concerning jails, crowded barracks, and transport ships. Hence, the fever has been called, hospital, jail, or ship fever, according with its place of origin.

The testimony of Dr. Jackson on the same head, is corroborative of what has been said. " I do not pretend to say," he observes, " that diseases arising from epidemic, *or even from common causes,* and which are not in their own nature contagious, *may not be so changed, by artificial circumstances,* as to assume a process, *which actually generates the matter of contagion.*"—Vol. i. p. 34. The same author adds, " It is known, *from undeniable testimonies of military history,*

that the camp or gastric fever of Autumn, though originating radically from an endemic cause, is readily converted into,
or rather with difficulty prevented from degenerating into the
hospital, or personally infectious fever of Winter." Pp. 31-2.

Dr. Johnson, in his book, on Air, p. 92, states, that a
typhus fever was generated on board the crowded transport
ships, which brought the army of Sir John Moore from
Corunna.

To give all the proof which has been furnished by authors,
would exceed the bounds of the present work. Every remarkable siege or extraordinary event, which collected crowds
of people in small confined places, whether at sea or on
shore, has furnished instances of this kind, as the writings of
ancient and modern historians have recorded.

Dr. Adams, although he denies the possibility of generating
contagion equivocally, allows " hospital fever may be excited
*by the accumulation of sick, whatever the nature of their
complaint may be*" (On Epidemics, p. 21); but according to
him, plague, hospital, jail, and yellow fevers, are not contagious. Dr. Bancroft, the other sceptic, as to the equivocal
generation of a contagion, believes plague to be " essentially
and specifically contagious," and styles typhus, the jail, or
contagious fever; but contests the opinion of Dr. Adams and
others with regard to its being ever excited by any thing except contagion itself. Yellow fever, according to him, is never
contagious under any circumstances; yet, at p. 314 of his
Essay, when giving an account of the epidemic yellow fever
of Barbadoes of 1647, which, he says, was " the earliest of
which we have any distinct account," adds, " about the time
when this fever prevailed, there had been a great and sudden
influx of inhabitants from England, in consequence of the
civil commotions at home, and of other causes. Indeed
*there never has been an extensively epidemic yellow fever in
the West Indies, without the previous arrival of considerable
numbers of persons from more temperate climates.* Hence,
times of *sickness* have *there* commonly been times of war."

Had the disease been always confined to the new comers on such occasions, Dr. B.'s inference in favour of climate and locality would have been conclusive ; but we shall afterwards shew that this *was never the case*. Barbadoes, in 1647, had been forty-two years settled, during which time, yellow fever had been unknown in that, the most healthy of all the islands in the West Indies ; nor had it appeared in any other place in that part of the world. All the strangers, who must have arrived from more temperate climates, escaped, *till some extraordinary circumstance, such as had long been known to excite pestilential diseases in other countries, occurred.* Then the disease is not confined to strangers ; for, according to Mr. Vines, one of Dr. B.'s own authorities, " *Many* who had began and almost finished great sugar works, who dandled themselves in their hopes, *were suddenly laid in the dust*, and their estates left unto strangers ;" these very strangers who, the passage quoted from the Doctor's essay would lead us to believe, were the only sufferers. Dr. B.'s observation, " there never has been an extensively epidemic yellow fever in the West Indies without the previous arrival of considerable numbers of persons *from more temperate climates*," is not quite correct. Two of the most celebrated and most extensive yellow fever epidemics on record, were cases where no persons had arrived *from more temperate climates.* The one appeared at Martinico, in 1686, soon after the arrival of a number of poor disappointed adventurers *from Siam, in the East Indies ;* the other at Grenada, in 1793, after the arrival of the ship Hankey, *from the Coast of Africa*, with a number of persons *under similar circumstances ;* and, perhaps the whole history of medicine, cannot furnish two instances where a contagion was more likely *to be generated and imported*, than these very cases. In what country, as well as the West Indies, have not times of sickness commonly been times of war ? But as we have not the smallest intention to detract from the merits of any author, particularly one so highly and justly distinguished as Dr. Bancroft, we think it but justice

I

to give his own words regarding typhus. " I believe," he says, " in the existence of a fever, *sui generis*, strictly contagious (unconnected with the exanthematous diseases), and, therefore, according to my view of the subject, derived exclusively from its own *specific cause*, or contagion. In this, which I consider as the only contagious fever, there are, I think, some varieties, but without any differences sufficient to form more than one species. The facts and reasons which have led me to this belief, will have been seen in the second part of this volume, at p. 104, et seq., *and they are sufficient, in my judgment, to outweigh all the great authorities to which they are opposed*, and render it absolutely incredible that any inanimate matters, even those excreted by living animals, should, by any natural or artificial decomposition and recomposition, ever acquire a power strictly contagious, or in other words, be enabled, like living animals and vegetables, to assimilate other matters to their own nature, and thus multiply and perpetuate their existence. Some writers of considerable reputation, sensible, perhaps, of this difficulty, have made a distinction between contagion and infection, and have ascribed the production of typhus fever, and some other diseases, to the latter. One of these writers, Doctor Adams, (in the quarto edition of his observations on Morbid Poisons, at p. 6,) after adopting this distinction, says of ' infectious diseases,' that they ' do not require for their production matter similar to their effects, but *may at any time be generated by crowding together the sick or wounded of any description.*' He then mentions ' hospital, prison, or ship fever, camp dysentery, and some peculiarly malignant ulcers,' as being infectious diseases ; adding that, ' though these diseases, when formed, *may produce their like effects in others*, yet we can always trace their origin *in causes different from their effects*.' That Dr. Adams, who is accustomed and qualified to reason, should have believed any thing so unphilosophical and incongruous, would have been incomprehensible to me, *if so many others had not discarded common sense* on the subject of contagion. To represent a disease which is *notoriously contagious*, and propagated by contagion, as capable of being also produced by other, and these very different means, is to multiply causes unnecessarily, and, therefore, unjustifiably; and, it moreover destroys the natural and just influence of causes upon their effects, by making the same disease result from very dissimilar causes." —*Essay*, pp. 498—502. The same author, at p. 104, the place he refers to in the above passage for his reasons, says, " Every thing which I have been able to discover or ascertain respecting the nature and properties of contagion, induces me to consider each of its several species as a peculiar morbid quality, or power, imparted to certain animal secretions, *in consequence of some particular, though unknown actions* excited in the living body when actually disordered by the very same species of contagion." The question, then, to be considered here, even according to Dr. B.'s own showing, is not whether dissimilar matters may, by decomposition and recomposition, generate a contagion without the body, *but whether such matters are capable of exciting, under any circumstances, that particular and unknown action in the living body which is necessary, in all cases, to impart the morbid quality to certain animal secretions, called contagion.* Now, that similar morbid actions are often excited in the animal system by dissimilar and even apparently opposite means, and that the body of a living animal has the power of assimilating different matters by actions peculiar to itself, are facts which we believe few physiologists or pathologists will deny. What the Doctor contends, therefore, at p. 105, appears to be false reasoning; he there observes, " If it were true that vegetable and animal matters, while decomposing or putrefying, could *de novo* generate contagion properly so called, *the species or varieties of contagion ought necessarily to have become as numerous and various as the matters so decomposing, and also as various as their relative proportions;*" but the Doctor might just as well assert, that the natural secretions of a living animal ought to keep pace with the number, proportion, and different kinds of food: according to this argument, the urine of a Gentoo should be different from that of a London Alderman ; the tears of a Hottentot, from those of an Esquimaux ; and the gastric juice of the peasant different from that of the peer. " Human existence ought, in such a case," the Doctor thinks, "to have become, with such additions to the other dangers which surround us, the most precarious, transient, and deplorable of all the works of creation." To this argument, all must assent ; it is, however, to be borne in mind that, although the contagions may be generated by dissimilar matters, they are also extremely liable to be destroyed, like all other known matters in a similar form, by a great number of other agents. Indeed, had they never been reproduced by dissimilar means, they must long ere this have become extinct ; for in most instances where Nature seems careful in preserving things from generation to generation, she has not left the matter to chance, but imparts to them either the quality of indestructibility by other agents, as in some kinds of inert matter, or certain inherent propensities, as in the case of animals and plants, to perpetuate their existence. Again, if we lay aside all the facts mentioned by authors, and which militate against Dr. B.'s theory, still the conclusions are irresistible : 1st. That no animal secretion could exist before the animal itself ; 2nd. That no morbid secretion is ever formed in the animal body in a state of health ; consequently, that all these morbid productions must have been once formed without causes similar to their effects, unless we can prove that man was first created in a state of disease.

Evidence of Contagion.

He who would aspire to the high character of a judge, must strictly observe certain rules in taking evidence, the propriety

of which will be plain to any one on the smallest reflection. If his object be to investigate truth, he is bound to
listen with patience to both sides of the question in dispute,
and to give credence to the testimony, according to the respectability, capacity, and opportunities for judging of the
witnesses. He must reject with scorn the evidence of any
witness who evinces a leaning to one side of the question,
whether that bias appear in his testimony or in his general
behaviour, and, for like reasons, he ought carefully to avoid
even the smallest appearance of favour or partiality in his
own conduct towards those he examines. All species of
tampering with the witnesses, by using threats or remon-
strances, by coaxing, wheedling, promise of fee or reward, &c.
are every way as inadmissible in taking real evidence, as the
Ottoman bowstring, or the thumb-screws of the Spanish
Inquisition. The last rule undoubtedly is never to allow
negative proof to outweigh positive and direct evidence, far
less to admit or receive the negative proof of one thing as
the positive proof of another. Any one who rejects these
simple rules in taking evidence, acts as a party, not as a
judge. He virtually, therefore, comes under the rules himself,
which direct us to receive his testimony, even as a witness,
with suspicion. The reasonableness of this last conclusion
must be evident on reflection ; for, supposing such a witness
really believes all he says to be true, his credence can only
be grounded on a conviction of one or two things, which
require first to be indisputably established by proof before his
testimony as to the point in dispute can be for a moment
listened to ; namely, his own superior talent and opportunities
for observation, or the total worthlessness and incapacity of
all those who have given contrary evidence ; and he must likewise judge of all that has been seen by others by what he
himself hath seen. In judging of the existence of a matter
like contagion, which Dr. Bancroft acknowledges can be
" neither seen, heard, nor felt," there must be many
sources of error ; and that man must possess something like

supernatural powers before he can justly arrogate to himself the exclusive privilege of positively deciding on its existence or non-existence. But would we lessen the difficulty by proceeding on the fallacious grounds he recommends (p. 94), by drawing important conclusions from negative proof, or by making partial appearances the criteria of general judgment? Would it be wise or safe to decide on the common occurrences of life, or on any of the established laws of Nature in this way? Would it not be more advisable to investigate contagion by the rule we judge of other matters, the existence of which are not susceptible of direct proof, that is by their effects? For instance, the question may be asked, is the sun a source of caloric or heat?—this question cannot be decided by direct demonstration. Caloric itself is invisible, untangible, imponderable, and unappreciable except by its effects. Nor have we direct proof of its being derived from the sun. When that luminary arises in the eastern horizon, the well-known effects of caloric are instantly perceived; as it approaches, the heat increases in proportion, and it declines again as the sun goes down or retires. When objects intervene and prevent the free passage of the calorific rays of the sun, the effects of heat are not felt beyond the obstructing media. If the rays be concentrated by a glass which allows of their being freely transmitted, the heat is prodigiously increased in power. This is deemed evidence sufficient that the sun is a source of heat.

Is measles a contagious disease? This is not susceptible of direct proof. No one ever saw the contagion of measles —no one ever weighed, or to his knowledge touched it. Like caloric, it is only appreciable by its effects; for we have no direct proof of contagion being derived from the body of a person labouring under measles. When such a person approaches near to one in health, the effects of contagion are instantly perceived on him by a sick smell. As both persons approach each other, the effects are increased in proportion. They are diminished as they retire from one another. If any body be placed between so as to obstruct the passage of the emanations from their source, the effects are not felt beyond the obstructing media. But these emanations can be collected and concentrated, so as to increase their effects to a prodigious degree. The proof then that contagion is derived from measles is just as conclusive as that heat is derived from the sun. Can the presence or quantity of caloric in a body be always perceived by its usual effects? No— caloric may be present in a body without its effects being perceptible. The same thing takes place in contagion. Are all persons alike sensible to caloric? No—some are more susceptible than others; so it happens in contagion. Can the latent caloric existing in a body be called into action by a change of circumstances? Yes—so can latent contagion in the animal system be excited. Are all inanimate bodies alike capable of conducting or transmitting caloric? No—some conduct and preserve it much better than others—this too with contagion. Does caloric spread from any given point in all directions with the same facility? No—it spreads in certain directions, and with greater or less rapidity in proportion to the quantity and quality of the combustible materials that happen to be present—so does contagion. If caloric has destroyed the inflammable materials which existed in a body by passing through it, is that body again capable of combustion? No—neither is a human body capable of being again infected with the same species of contagion. Has the atmosphere much influence in regulating or affecting caloric? Certainly—so the matter stands with contagion. Thus, then, the method of judging by induction and by analogy, may often lead us to the most correct and certain conclusions. What would be the results were we to adopt the method by allowing negative to outweigh positive evidence. Crowding, filth, nastiness, intercourse and communication with those labouring under contagious diseases, do not always engender or propagate contagion. We have given some satisfactory reasons why they do not. But we beg to remind

Dr. Bancroft, who lays so much stress on negative evidence, and who seems fond of drawing comparisons between animal generation and that of contagion, that sexual intercourse does not always succeed in propagating the human species.* Many melancholy instances might be found almost in every parish where it has failed. Nor are the annals of medicine *barren* on this head. Several bulky tomes might easily be filled from well-authenticated sources. Similar exceptions may likewise be found in the general laws of Nature.

Intercourse and communication with the sick is the grand test by which we judge of the nature of a malady. If a disease be increased when intercourse with the sick is increased, and diminished in frequency when such intercourse is lessened, surely that disease will be best prevented by cutting off communication with the sick. He who acted on this principle could not be accused of either the ignorance or credulity of the simple Otaheitians, who carry their belief in contagion so far as to avoid the hump-backed or bandy-legged European, lest their own handsome persons should become similarly deformed by holding communication for a short time with them.† Those who witness the slow and gradual progress of a disease proceeding from individual to individual, and multiplying itself according to the degree of intercourse with those labouring under it, will act wisely not to stop and enquire whether the wind is in the North or in the South; whether the moon is in her first quarter, or in her wane; whether the heat be as high as 70° of Fahrnheit, or below 50°;

* Some cases are recorded where the female conceived after a lapse of twenty-seven years.

† An instance of this kind is said to have occurred during the visit of Vancouver. One of his sailors being on shore was followed, as usual, by the curious multitude. Having a river to ford, the sailor pulled up his trowsers; the natives were panic struck to discover that his legs were deformed, and hesitated to cross the river lest they should catch the infection. He was immediately forsaken, and left to pursue his walk alone. These islanders go so far as to say that a ship passing the island has sent a disease amongst them.—*See Turnbull's Voyages.*

or whether there happen to have been thirty days drought, or moist weather, or much rain.   On the contrary, they will include all distempers in the class of contagious diseases which have the power of propagating themselves, *under certain circumstances,* from the diseased to the healthy ; " whether they are communicable only by a specific matter, as small-pox, measles, cow-pox and lues, or are also generated by other causes, as typhus ; whether they affect the same person only once, as small-pox, or repeatedly, as lues ; whether the matter which appears to be the immediate means of propagation be considered as an excretion or secretion ; whether it acts only when applied in substance, as cow-pox, or through the medium of the atmosphere, as in *chin-cough,* or in both ways, as in small-pox ; whether it be visible, as in cow-pox and small-pox, or invisible, as in chin-cough and measles ; and whatever its nature and chemical composition may be whether acid, alkaline, or neither ; whether contagion be, considered as a property common to several kinds of matter, or a peculiar principle capable of imparting the property to these kinds of matter."—Vide *Ed. Med. Journ.* vol. i.

It matters not to the sufferer, whether the agent by which he suffers be baptised a contagion or an infection, an emanation or exhalation, a secretion or excretion, a principle or a property, a miasm or an effluvium, an atom, element or particle, a specific, septic or antisepic, the fact is the same by whatever name it may be called.   It is a morbid poison, which depends for its existence on intercourse and communication.   Nor would it be advisable for any one to lose much time at first in making scrupulous genealogical inquiries concerning the birth, parentage, or pedigree of this mischievous progeny.   For whether the child be come to the full time, or be only an abortion ; whether it be a hybrid,*

---

* Dr. Adams who, as we have seen, believes in the equivocal generation of hospital fevers, which Dr. Bancroft allows is " *notoriously contagious,*" observes " it has been said that no combination of them (cow-pox and small-pox matter) will ever produce a hybrid disease.   I am not fond of

a bastard, or a child lawfully begotten; and whatever its
relationship to others of a similar kind may be, uncle, aunt,
cousin-german, or one twenty times removed, are all questions of secondary importance; his malevolent propensities
is the first thing to provide against. And, whether he present
himself in the usual form, or assume some more questionable
shape; whether he be sober and regular in his habits, or
whimsical, capricious, and treacherous in his proceedings;
still we must never be off our guard; and, in all cases of
doubt, it is better to act on the principle of danger from
intercourse and communication, than allow ourselves to fall
into a state of passive and misplaced security.

Sphere of Contagion.

" By the knowledge of the present day," says Dr. Rollo, "contagion can only arise and spread under absolute inattention
and neglect." No one, who has made himself acquainted with
the labours of Haygarth, Perceval, Currie, Clark, &c., can
doubt the truth of this assertion. Before their time, physicians entertained very vague notions as to the distance to which
contagion might extend from its source, some believing that
the infection of small-pox may extend to the distance of
thirty miles (See *Haygarth's Letter to Dr. Perceval*, p. 87),
others to the distance of 1,500 feet (*Clark's Papers*, vol. ii.
p. 89). Dr. Haygarth first started a doctrine, about sixty
years ago, which was directly contrary to the most respectable
opinions that then prevailed; and, in a letter to Dr. Clark,
published in October, 1802, he says, " Yet, during the long
time which has since elapsed, thirty years, not a single fact
has been produced to contradict my conclusions, that the in-

adopting a term which may produce further altercation for want of a
proper definition, but that the diseases may be confounded, that is, that
the laws peculiar to one may occasionally influence the other, will appear
by the following registers."—See *Morb. Poisons*, p. 16.

fection of the small-pox never extends beyond the house which contains the poison, so as to be communicated to any person in an adjoining house, or even in the street, to which the doors and windows open from the pestilential chamber." *(Ibid.)* Professor Waterhouse, who had supported, in some of his letters, the opinion that small-pox might infect at a great distance, *chiefly on the authority of others*, became a proselyte to Dr. H.'s doctrine, and he asserted publicly his change of opinion, affirming that for six months, when the small-pox had been epidemical at Boston, he observed no instance where the distemper was conveyed by the wind to a distance. " In the family of a poor woman," Dr. H. says, " in Handbridge, a suburb of Chester, two of her children were attacked by the small-pox, and one of them died. I promised her a reward of ten shillings, if she would observe *the rules of prevention*, which require nothing but cleanliness and se- paration. Except a boy, who had been in the sick chamber before the directions were given, not a single child caught the disease, though two were liable to it, even at the next door, and not fewer than twenty-six in the near neighbour- hood. The girl who died, was, for a fortnight, during the day, in the room to which the outer door immediately opens ; the path runs as close as possible to the door where the children constantly passed, and often played."—*Inquiry*, p. 93.

" A young man, came from a distance with a fever upon him, it proved to be the small-pox, and of a confluent kind, of which he died on the 28th or 29th day. He lodged in Selburgh, which cannot be more than three yards broad. He lay up one pair of stairs, but at the head of them there was no door, the foot of the stairs is close to the door which opens into the street; the house where he was, being exceed- ing small, and he a very lusty man, there was not a particle of air in any of the rooms, but what was impregnated with the contagion, as might be discovered by the smell. Upon going into the house, the offensive stench struck one imme- diately ; and, as the door was a bad one, I am pretty confident, might have been perceived before it was opened. No particular precautions were used by the uninfected, except by keeping out of the house; the nurses were desired to wash the dirty clothes, and to carry away all discharges, &c., from the patient, at proper hours. The small-pox had not been epidemical at Selburgh for upwards of seven years. Some of the next-door neighbours had not had the distemper, nor great numbers of children who had passed through the streets every day, yet not one caught the infection."—*Satch*, p. 193.

On the two former and many other similar facts, the Small-pox Society at Chester was established. In one short comprehensive sentence, the extensive and uniform experience of the society is explicitly stated. " During the last six years, from 1778 till 1784, few weeks have elapsed without positive proofs that the infectious influence did not extend to the adjoining houses."—*Inquiry*, p. 184. " Several hundred double rewards were given to persons who had merited them, by a faithful and successful observation of the rules of prevention. In regard to the facts related in the proceedings of the society, it should be observed that they are ascertained with a great degree of authority, by a committee consisting of all the medical, and many other intelligent members of the society. The poor people who claim these rewards, come regularly before these gentlemen every month. The double reward is not to be obtained, except by those who have preserved *all* their neighbours and acquaintance from the infection. Besides a written certificate from their inspector, they are examined in the presence of others, who have in some instances transgressed the rules, and whose reward is consequently diminished; these would complain of injustice, if there was any pretence for complaint.—*Inquiry*, p. 182.

We have given the above facts regarding the small distance to which small-pox can be conveyed through the atmosphere, only as a specimen of innumerable instances that might be added of a similar kind. Although the very limited sphere of this fatal disease has been perfectly ascertained for more than half a century, it has not always been acted upon, as we shall soon be able to demonstrate. We have found many respectable medical men, who either did not know it or did not believe it, and to whom the works of Haygarth, Perceval, Clark, Currie, &c. &c., were only known by name. If vague notions be entertained by some of the profession regarding contagion, it cannot be expected that the public in general can be better informed; consequently, small-pox, even at the present day, is sometimes allowed to commit its dreadful ravages on suffering humanity, without due and vigorous measures of prevention being persevered in. The following melancholy proof of this fact lately fell under our own notice.

In the Spring of 1830, the small-pox was introduced into the Island of Malta, as was believed, by his Majesty's ship Asia, a circumstance which could not fail of spreading great alarm throughout the whole population, native as well as European. The grounds for this alarm will appear when it is stated, that vaccination, though recommended and promoted by the Government, by medical men, both native and European, and even by the clergy of different persuasions, had been here, as in England and many other countries of Europe, much neglected. It is not an easy task to rouse a people into a sense of duty where danger and suffering have been long absent: the narrow streets and crowded population of the towns in Malta; the great number of populous villages, and the perpetual intercourse kept up between them and the capital and with each other; the vicinity of the garrisons, hospitals, and charitable and other public institutions, to some of the most crowded parts of the city; the prodigious number of poor in every part of the town and country; the unrestrained mode in which they ask for charity in the streets, markets, and even churches; the great proportion of pauper clergy, monks, &c., and the constant intercourse between them and the laity; the habit, in Catholic countries, of visiting the sick and the dying; the alarm excited by the host, and constant tolling of the death-bell; the mixture of all ranks in the churches, their taste for masquerades, feasting and fasting; the anxiety evinced by the sick and convalescent to be present at all religious ceremonies; the presence of a large fleet with the number of ships in the harbour, and the great traffic and intercourse by boats; altogether presented such a field for the spreading of a contagious disease like small-pox, which we believe, has seldom, if ever been excelled. The season was, also, favourable. What then but the most determined exertions of the government, the medical profession, the clergy, and even of the people, could possibly have averted the direful consequences which followed. Vaccination was practised as a means of prevention, and recommended by the clergy; two wards of the civil hospital were set apart for the reception of cases, one for men, and one for women, these were a little apart from the other wards; a regular report of cases was kept by the Police; the General directed the necessary precautions to be used for the protection of the military, and Vice Admiral Sir Pulteney Malcolm, for that of the fleet, so far all was right; but we never could learn that any vigorous and well digested plan had been adopted for purifying and washing the clothes, bedding, furniture, and dwellings of the sick poor, much less of those who had had communication with them; without this, every effort to suppress the disease, was sure to prove fruitless. At our arrival in Malta, in June, from Algiers (where we had been detained two months, to attend the families of the British Consul General and Vice Consul), the disease was committing dreadful ravages amongst the native population, who, being the poorest of the community, could not but be more exposed to infection. As ignorance and prejudice prevailed more amongst them, it was besides greatly to be feared, that the practice of vaccination had been more neglected, consequently, that a much larger proportion of the natives were susceptible, their constitutions being wholly unprotected, either by vaccination or by a previous attack of small-pox. An opportunity so favorable for observation was not to be lost; we therefore, spent much of our time in making inquiries. With this view we visited the sick in their own wretched abodes, as also the patients in the small-pox hospital. One of the first patients we saw was a fine Maltese boy, about ten years of age; the scene was truly distressing. The house in which he was, consisted of one apartment, with only one window. On an indifferent-looking bed, lay the unconscious victim in a moribund state; the eye was fixed and almost lifeless; the face was covered with innumerable pustules, which had now assumed a black hue; the muscles of the lower jaw had lost their power, and thus afforded a view of the mouth, tongue, and throat, all in a similar state of disease; in short, little signs of life remained, except now and then, at awful intervals of time, a convulsive heave of the chest and apparently the last effort at inspiration. Many people of both sexes and different ages stood in silence around the bed, as if anxious to watch the soul's departure, and gather the last dregs of poison from his corrupted and mortal body. On trying to depart from the house, we found the passage much obstructed by crowds of people, chiefly women and children. A loud-sounding bell was heard as if at a distance, and also the sound of several human voices chanting a hymn; it was the approach of the host to the boy we had just left. This procession was followed by a crowd of the same class of persons, who, with the others, stood near the house till the religious ceremony was finished.

It is fearful to contemplate the number of persons that must have come in close contact with the contagion of small-pox, even from this single patient. Those persons who stood closely round the bed, and who had remained no doubt a considerable time in the infected atmosphere of the sick apartment, must have mixed, first with the priests and persons within the house, then with those around the door, and

these again with others. But to trace contagion from individual to individual in such a scene, would be as impossible
as to trace the air which had before filled the lungs of each,
so that many persons might be eventually infected who had
never been conscious of coming in contact with the cause
of disease, and some persons might infect others though not
liable to it themselves.

At an interview we had with Sir Frederick Hankey, who
had on another occasion shewn us some marks of kindness,
we took the liberty of representing these defects in the mode
of prevention. We likewise strongly urged the necessity of
adopting some more vigorous measures, and we offered to
prove the practicability of arresting the progress of the disease by actual experiment under our own immediate inspection, for which we neither asked nor expected any reward.
An hour was appointed next day to meet and confer with
Dr. Gravagne, the medical officer of police and quarantine,
on the subject; but it unfortunately happened, that this
gentleman, like many well-meaning and even well-informed
persons on other medical subjects in our own country, had
adopted the opinion, that the contagion of small-pox was
capable of diffusion through the air to a considerable distance from its source, so as to prove infectious; consequently, that all our proposed plans for suppressing the
disease must be ineffectual, and only give rise to trouble
and expence. In support of his opinion, Dr. Gravagne
stated, that since the opening of the small-pox hospital, the
disease had spread much in its neighbourhood, though no
person but the nurses and medical attendants had been
allowed to enter its walls. In our turn, we endeavoured to
convince our opponent, that the increase of small-pox in the
neighbourhood of the hospital was by no means occasioned
by the diffusion of the contagion in the air, but from the
intercourse of the sick people's friends with the people who
lived in its neighbourhood. Sometimes the greater part of a
family was admitted into the small-pox wards at the same

time, and their friends anxious to learn their fate made enquiries in the houses in the vicinity. It was surely, therefore, nothing surprising if people just arrived from the contaminated dwellings, a little before left by the sick, conveyed the contagion to the houses they entered, and made their enquiries, seeing that no precautions had been taken to prevent an occurrence so likely to happen. Had this subject been discussed in the presence of a medical committee appointed for the purpose, it is very likely our arguments would have prevailed, as many of the respectable medical men were of our way of thinking; as, without such support, we could not expect to succeed, it was thought advisable to yield. It is proper to state, that Sir Frederick Hankey was not present at this conference.

The following is a copy of the official report of the cases of small-pox in the Island of Malta, between the 17th of March, and the 31st of July, 1830, which was given us by our friend, Dr. Gravagne, when we left Malta.

Total number affected...................... 2691
Not vaccinated 1804
Supposed vaccinated 851
Who had before small-pox 42
DEATHS.—Total number ascertained 327
Not vaccinated 276
Supposed vaccinated 27
Who had before small-pox............... 4
                    (Signed)   D. GRAVAGNE.

The small-pox was still spreading rapidly when this report was made ; but we had no opportunity of learning its after-progress, as we sailed for Tripoli, Tunis, Algiers, Oran, soon after.

Malta affords some facilities to the suppression of a contagion like small-pox. 1st. The inhabitants have been long familiarised with quarantine and other means of prevention ; and, as they have more than once suffered dreadfully from

K

their neglect, all classes must be well aware of the expediency, nay, absolute necessity of adopting them. 2nd. His Excellency, General Ponsonby, the present governor, Sir Frederick Hankey, and the other members of the British Government, are deservedly popular: what would require compulsion with some governments, might be done with persuasion by them. 3rd. The people are much under the influence of their numerous clergy, who have uniformly been most faithful and zealous in forwarding the views of Government. 4th. The Maltese themselves are a sober, orderly, industrious, and tractable people. 5th. The majority of the medical practitioners in Malta are well informed; and great care has been taken to improve the course of medical education in their school of medicine. Lastly, the police and quarantine establishments, which are very extensive, are both admirably regulated. Perhaps, no place in the world possesses more advantages in this respect than Malta; for not only different parts of the island, but the different towns, and even parts of towns, might easily be insulated by a few soldiers, and kept from all communication with each other. The large military force, the mildness of the climate, the practice of bathing and sleeping in the open air, the facilities for encampment, &c., all contribute in rendering the task of prevention more easy. As to the mode of prevention which ought to have been persevered in on the present occasion, it can all be comprehended in four words—vaccination, ventilation, separation, and cleanliness. The narrow sphere of other contagions has been as well ascertained as that of small-pox.

"I have had occasion to know," says the late Professor Gregory, of Edinburgh, in a letter to Dr. Clark, "that many well-meaning and really sensible people, merely from being unacquainted with the subject, have conceived a fever-ward or fever-hospital, to be the very reverse of what it really is— a great magazine of the most pestilential contagion—*when in truth, it is the best preventive of the formation of many such receptacles and sources of contagion.*"

The Royal Infirmary of Edinburgh stands in a *fully* inhabited part of the city, and it is an asylum for those labouring under fever as well as under other diseases. Between the window of the clinical ward appropriated to the women, as well as of a *fever ward,* and those of a neighbouring house, thirty feet do not intervene. These wards have windows almost constantly open on each side to the above house, and to others, yet no instance has occurred, within the recollection of Dr. Duncan, Professor of Medicine, which extends more than thirty years back, of infection being conveyed to any of these houses. So little apprehension, indeed, have the inhabitants of Edinburgh, of the Infirmary being a cause of diffusing contagion to the neighbourhood, that a piece of ground (opposite the College, and closely adjoining to one of the fever-wards), being put up to auction, although it only furnishes sites for five houses, and in some points is not more than forty or fifty feet from the fever-wards, lately sold for the amazing sum of £11,000. This sale took place about the year 1800; consequently, the narrow sphere of contagion has been known in Edinburgh for nearly sixty years.

Dr. Wardell, a physician in the army, observes: " I was early led to think the influence of contagious matter producing fever was confined within narrow bounds, and I as soon thought I perceived the importance of cleanliness and ventilation in preventing its generation, and, when existing, in weakening its power, if not immediately destroying it. I could, in almost innumerable instances, shew, that in hospitals, even in such temporary incommodious buildings as an army is often compelled to take up with for regimental ones, when properly conducted, fever cases have been admitted with perfect safety to the other patients of the hospital, and that so invariably, that for some years past, no hesitation whatever has been entertained on the admission of them. I could likewise shew that, in many instances (and I know of no one to the contrary), by strict attention to personal cleanliness, ventilation, and fumigation of the barrack-rooms, the fumes of fever of malignant character have been almost invariably extinguished. This was the case with the 31st Regiment of Foot, the 14th Light Dragoons, and 32nd Foot. The two former were at the time in the barracks at Canterbury, and the other at Ashford. During the prevalence of the fevers in these regiments, there did not occur one instance of the communication of fever in the respective hospitals, while the fever patients were accommodated in separate wards.

" In times of sickness like those I have mentioned, we found great difficulty in procuring proper accommodation for the sick soldiers; and, perhaps, in no place do greater apprehensions prevail than in Canterbury. The clergy there, supported by a few alarmists of the faculty, had almost shut every door against us; and all reasoning and remonstrance were in vain, till I referred them to a matter subjected to their own observation or personal enquiry, to ascertain the truth of. At this time there were three temporary hospitals in Canterbury; they were hired dwelling-houses, *situated in the public streets,* and in contact with inhabited houses on each side; two of them had been employed for regimental hospitals six or seven years, and the other about four. I do not recollect that any one of them was, for any time together, exempt from cases of fever; yet, never in a single instance was a fever, or indeed any contagious febrile complaint, communicated to the inhabitants of the adjoining houses. This was a matter keenly looked into; and glad, I believe, the enquirers would have been, could they have detected a single instance, even of an ambiguous nature, to support their opposition and their prejudices; but the fact *was incontrovertible."—Letter to Dr. Clark.*

The experience of Dr. Lind on this point, was greater, perhaps, than that of any single person. It corroborates what has been stated—he says, " In Haslar Hospital, where, during war, the number of contagious diseases is greater than can be expected in any private institution, the fever-wards are in each wing, connected by a piazza to the rest of the hospital, and employ without inconvenience the common kitchen, wash-house, and other offices. Observation does not warrant the apprehension that contagion might be communicated to the infirmary, from the windows of the fever-wards, through the medium of the external air; with due ventilation and cleanliness, contagion would seldom be considerable in these wards, and in the free air beyond very confined limits, *even strong contagion would lose its power of exciting disease.*" A remarkable instance of this occurred to Dr. L. during his attendance on Forton Prison, in 1780. In March and April, near 3,000 prisoners were received at Forton ; 1769 Spaniards, and 1206 French, and in successive detachments most of them forwarded to other prisons. Forton, in the meantime, became sickly; for above three weeks it was very crowded ; afterwards the number of prisoners was reduced to nearly 800 Spanish, and 200 French.

The Spanish prisoners brought with them a typhus fever, which, during the crowded state of Forton, spread both to the prison and hospital. The contagion was so strong that, at the expiration of ten days, of *twenty-seven* of the Spanish prisoners employed to attend their sick, only *one* had escaped the fever: out of twenty-three nurses and labourers, twenty-two were either sick or dead : the barber and four interpreters in succession, there being only one interpreter allowed at a time upon the books. The contagion continued seventeen weeks, and *absorbed among the Spanish all other diseases.* During that period, 795 Spaniards were admitted into the hospital, including re-admissions, and 156 died. The French were confined in the same general prison with the Spanish, were lodged at night in separate wards, but used through the day the same common airing-ground, kitchen, and offices. From a national aversion, the Spaniards would not permit a Frenchman to associate with them. Thus situated, the French in a great measure escaped the contagion ; few of them had fevers, and the fevers of those few were slight. During the whole period of the contagion, only *five* French prisoners died. At the same time 229 Americans were confined in another part of Forton prison : they were not allowed any intercourse with the other prisoners, but the hospital which contained the sick Spaniards ranged along one side of their airing-ground, separated only by a narrow causeway, and had, near the ceiling of each ward, ventilators opening towards their airing-ground. These Americans remained perfectly free from contagion : not one American died during the fever months, in which the contagion prevailed so severely among the Spaniards.

Dr. Saunders, after having been a physician to a large hospital (Guy's) for upwards of thirty years, concurs with Drs. Haygarth and Clark in their opinion, and he adds, " a dispensary physician, who visits the dirty confined habitations of the poor is always in danger, while the same attention in an airy well-ventilated atmosphere is accompanied with little or no danger."

Dr. George Pearson agrees, and says, " that infectious fevers may be admitted into any hospital with perfect safety to the other patients, where there are wards appropriated exclusively for the reception of such diseases, and where ventilation and cleanliness are daily attended to, *is a matter established beyond a doubt.*"

Mr. Pearson, of the Lock Hospital, having been much troubled by patients introducing contagion of fever amongst the other patients of that establishment, was forced to have recourse to separate fever-wards, as a means of prevention. These wards had an immediate communication with the wards of the hospital; nevertheless, not a single instance had occurred for ten years, in which a fever had been communicated to any person in the hospital, nor had a single patient died of fever since the opening of the fever-wards. To the above testimonies, I still add, says Dr. Clark, the evidence of Dr. Rollo, Surgeon-General to the Royal Hospital at Woolwich, where the wards, though numerous, are small, and where those allotted for contagious fevers are only separated from others by a partition. " A patient with his clothes, admitted with an *infectious disease*, having undergone the washing and cleaning of his person, *and the lodgment of his clothes in the oven to be baked,* then fumigated and scoured, is put into a separate ward, or into one with a patient having a similar disease. All intercourse is prevented, except what is indispensible, by a sentinel placed on the outside of the door of the gallery. By these simple means, invariably prosecuted, infection does not spread in the hospital." Out of the whole number of patients admitted during five years, being 7526—381 laboured under fevers, of whom seventeen died ; and as only one in thirty-five died, during this period, out of the whole number of patients admitted under all diseases, a remarkable proof is thus afforded, that the admission of patients under fevers into *separate* and *distinct* wards, although even in the same hospital, does not add to its insalubrity.—See a *Short Account of the Artillery Hospital, at Woolwich, by Dr. Rollo,* pp. 73 and 116.

Dr. Cleghorn, of Glasgow, in a letter to Dr. Clark, dated July, 1802, says, " If the public shall not be convinced by the very ample evidence adduced by you, I fear my testimony will avail nothing. Be this, however, as it may, I do not hesitate to maintain that, by proper care, fevers might be nearly extirpated, and that no plan seems so proper for the purpose as fever-wards or houses properly managed. These never did nor never can become sources of contagion to infirmaries or neighbourhoods, unless, like the old Hôtel de Dieu in Paris, they be constructed on the worst possible plan, or were to be managed entirely by knaves and fools."

A military hospital has subsisted in Vine Lane, Newcastle, since the 16th December, 1801. The hospital is one of the best houses in that lane, where the buildings are continued in a line. At the time it was opened, a contagious fever was prevalent amongst the soldiers. One room or ward in this house was set apart for fevers exclusively. There was only the staircase between it and the entrance into the other wards; "there have been six patients," says the Surgeon, "at one time in the fever-ward, all extremely ill, and the other wards at the same time completely full with patients labouring under other complaints; yet, I can with great truth assert, that since the above period (viz. from December 16th, 1801, to July 1st, 1802), there was not one man in any of the other wards seized with any symptoms of fever."

Dr. Lind asserts, that he never himself found the least symptom of infection, although for several years he attended persons labouring under contagious diseases—that in eighteen months, only *five* persons died out of more than *one hundred* constantly employed as nurses; of these one died through a decay of nature; one had been an irregular drunken man; one was not treated as directed; and the other two were victims to their own indiscretion, having concealed under their beds, the clothes from persons violently affected." Whereas, at Forton prison, where ventilation, cleanliness, and other modes of prevention could not be so well attended to as in Haslar Hospital, we have seen that, in the short space of ten days, out of twenty-seven nurses, only one had escaped the fever; that out of twenty-three nurses and labourers, twenty-two were either sick or dead; and that the barber and four interpreters, had been seized in succession.

Sir William Watson, M.D. informed Dr. Haygarth, that in St. Thomas's Hospital, Drs. Akenside, Russel, Grieve, and Mr. Waren, surgeon, all of St. Thomas's, fell victims to the hospital fever, from having received the infection *in the consulting room.* According to Dr. Woodville, two other physicians of the same hospital, namely, Drs. Watkinson and Keir, and one of Guy's, Dr. Munckley, died of the same disease. Besides these, three physicians, and a medical student of one of the largest hospitals in London, died within the space of eight years of malignant fevers. If so many physicians fell victims to contagion in a few years, what must have yeen the mortality in the crowded wards of these and other hospitals in the metropolis, notwithstanding the restriction against the reception of infectious diseases. From what has been advanced, it will appear that the true and only certain way to secure hospitals and infirmaries from the contagion of fever, is to prevent its progress, and to exterminate it at the habitations of the poor.* Those who may wish to examine more evidence as to the narrow sphere of contagion, may peruse the papers collected by Dr. Clark, where, in addition to the above, they will find a host of evidence, including the distinguished testimonies of Hunter, Heberden, Willan, Beddoes, Baillie, Farquhar, Milman, Gartshore, Woodville, Lettsom, Dimsdale, Latham, Hamilton, Blane, Gilchrist, Campbell, Falconer, Bradley, Marcet, Horne, Cruickshanks, &c. &c. all on the same side.

The two following instances regarding scarlet fever deserve to be added. " Very lately the scarlet fever and sore throat appeared in a large boarding-school in this town (Newcastle). Six young ladies received the infection, probably from the same source. I was called to the first the moment she was taken ill, and I suspected her case would turn out scarlet

---

* A Report of the Medical Committee of the Metropolis, signed by Drs. Cooke, Willan, Stanger, Murray, Farquhar, Gartshore, Latham, and Lettsom, contains the following :—" From the experience of Chester, Manchester, Waterford, and other places, where houses for the reception of persons in fever have been established, we are satisfied that the number of contagious fevers has been greatly diminished, not only in town, but in the very district and neighbourhood where houses of recovery have been situated. From this circumstance, therefore, as well as from our own knowledge and the statement of those who have the best means of observation, we are of opinion, that the proper and necessary regulations for the internal management of the house in Gray's Inn-Lane-road being adopted, there will be no reasonable ground of apprehension on the part of the neighbouring inhabitants. On the contrary, we believe there will be much less danger of the atmosphere in that neighbourhood being infected by the proposed House of Recovery, *than there now is in the populous districts of the town from the prevalence of fever in workhouses, or in the habitations of the poor.*"

fever. The young lady, her clothes and bedding, were taken into a separate room, and I gave directions that the same measures should be followed with any other person in the house who might be seized with the slightest feverish symptom. In the course of a few days, the remaining five took the disease; one of whom died. My first patient continued in the boarding-school for above a week, the others only a few days, till lodgings out of the house could be procured. By following the rules of prevention, the disease did not spread to any more of the young ladies, or to any other person in the boarding-school, although it contained upwards of fifty." Dr. Clark adds, " in order to shew that I have not recommended a practice that I do not follow in my own family, and with my own respected friends, I beg leave to mention the following circumstance : My daughter lodged in a boarding-school in this town (Newcastle), where one of her young companions was seized with the scarlet fever. I did not take her home, because I knew rules of prevention would be strictly followed. The young lady who sickened was taken out of the house by the gentleman who attended her, and the disease made no further progress.

" Dr. Currie of Liverpool, had two daughters at the school first mentioned. The youngest was the person who first took the disease: his eldest daughter continued in the house during her illness. When Dr. Currie was informed of the circumstances, and of the measures that were taken to prevent the spreading of contagion, notwithstanding he had formerly lost a child in the same disease, he was perfectly satisfied, and desired her to remain at school.

" Dr. Perceval too had a daughter at the same school, who went to a gentleman's house in the country soon after the fever broke out. Miss Perceval, at the very time Miss Currie was ill of the fever, came to visit her sister. I gave it as my opinion, that she would be as safe at this school as in any house of the town, because I knew that every rule of prevention would be strictly followed. After staying two nights, she went to visit her sister, and after remaining two days, both returned to the boarding-school. I wrote to Dr. Perceval immediately, informing him of every particular: he was perfectly satisfied with the means taken, and his daughter still remains at the boarding-school. Such facts as these require no comment."

In April, 1779, Master Plumbe was attacked in a dangerous degree with a scarlet fever and sore throat in the house of his school-master at Chester. There were at this time thirty-seven young gentlemen, boarders in the family, most of whom, it is highly probable, were disposed to receive this dangerous contagion. The patient's chamber was situated *in the middle of the house*, at the landing of the first pair of stairs. All the scholars went close past his door several times a day. At this season, Winchester and several other large schools in England, sent home, and dispersed their scholars on account of this distemper, which had alarmingly spread among them. Dr. Haygarth, fully aware of the narrow sphere of variolous contagion, directed the rules of prevention to be placed on the patient's door in this case. The event fully justified his hopes; though all the thirty-seven scholars remained in the same house during the whole disease, yet not one of them was infected.—*Sketch*, p. 347. In October, 1778, out of forty young ladies at a boarding-school in Chester, all but four had scarlet fever; twelve very severely, and two most dangerously. "This comparative statement of facts," says Dr. H., "shows, beyond all reasonable doubt, to what a little distance from the poison the infectious miasms extend, and that *the rules of prevention* are in this respect fully adequate to their purpose."—*Ibid.*

In the year 1808, a typhus fever broke out in his Majesty's ships Stately and Nassau, then off the Coast of Denmark, which affected a considerable proportion of the crews, and proved fatal to about forty men in each ship. The berths on both sides of the cock-pit of the Nassau were full of young gentlemen at the time the fever appeared, as well as during the continuance of the ship at sea. Many of those living on the starboard side were seized with fever long before a single case occurred in the one opposite, although the distance between the cabins is very short, and a frequent communication was kept up between them. The good effects of free air were very striking ; the purser and surgeon who slept in the cockpit, both had it. Those sleeping in the ward-room cabins suffered less, and the captain above escaped it entirely. We cannot speak more positively, as we give the above particulars from recollection only.

Differences of Contagion.

Although the contagions possess certain properties, which are sufficiently common to distinguish them as a class, yet each has some individual pecularities; and, in some instances, several of them agree in certain points, while they differ materially in others. The qualities they have in common are— 1st. They are all increased by intercourse and communication with the sick, each producing its like in the sound person who has been exposed. 2nd. All of them may be prevented by separation, ventilation, cleanliness, and other means.

They differ, 1st. *In their origins*—some being derived from the brute creation, as vaccine matter from the cow and horse;* hydrophobia from the canine tribe. Several are peculiar to the human species, and do not affect brutes—brutes may, however, carry contagion from a sick to a well person, though not susceptible of it themselves. 2nd. *In their durations*—some of them (as the acute or febrile contagious diseases), are limited in their course to a short period only, within which the constitution resumes the healthy action or

---

* As there is no other instance of one contagion destroying the susceptibility to another, some believe small-pox and cow-pox had the same origin.

sinks under the disorder. The diseases caused by other contagions, as itch, venereal disease, &c., are longer in duration,
and are sometimes not susceptible of spontaneous cure, or one
unassisted by art. 3rd. *In the stage of the disease by which
they are produced.*—Hooping-cough is probably contagious
for a longer time than any other contagious disease ; plague
longer than small-pox or cow-pox ; typhus than yellow fever.
All acute contagious diseases, generate contagion of greater
power before than after their crisis. No body, if properly
cleaned, is infectious after death ; local as well as general
death destroys the creative process. 4th. *In the forms they
assume.*—Where the temperature of the atmosphere is never
sufficiently low, some contagions will assume a permanent
gaseous form. Where the temperature never ranges above
a certain degree, others will always assume a palpable form.
In some instances, the same contagion may exist in both
forms at the same time—in the same way that part of the
water rises into the atmosphere, and part remains in a fluid
form, at a time when the thermometer indicates the same degree of heat. On this account the contagions likewise differ.
5th. *In their sphere of action.*—All contagions are limited in
their power to a narrow sphere. Gaseous contagions operate
in confined atmospheres at a short distance from their source ;
contagion capable of existing only in a palpable form requires
contact. Those which assume both forms, operate both by
near approach to the sick and by contact. 6th. *In their
power of resisting other agents.*—Some are destroyed by cold,
others dissipated by heat : none of them can maintain an
independent existence, or retain their power of propagation
for any length of time, if exposed to the atmosphere. We want
further experiments to ascertain their respective powers in
this way. The length of time which variolous matter exposed to the air retains its contagious quality, depends on
its superficies. Spread thin upon glass, it sometimes disap-
points the inoculator at the end of twenty days, though not
generally : it has sometimes succeeded in communicating the

disease, even when diffused over a large surface, at the end of
seventy-three days; but this is not common. The instance
in which Dr. Currie, of Liverpool, found variolous matter to
retain its infectious quality longest, was the following : " On
the 2nd of February, 1792," he says, " he took a considerable quantity of this matter on a piece of window-glass, keeping it as much together as its fluidity would admit. It was
exposed immediately to a stream of air, and the surface was
speedily dry. On the 2nd of March following, upon moist-
ening a portion of it with a little water, he inoculated three
patients, and all with success. In the course of the Summer,
he inoculated with another portion of it, previously liquified
by the addition of warm water, and with success as before.
On the 20th of July, 1793, he again used a portion of the
same matter in the same way, and again with success ; but
this success was long doubtful, and it was not till the twenty-
second day after the operation that the patient sickened ; he
tried the same matter in June, 1794, when it entirely failed."
He adds, " it is now by me, and is not mouldy, nor any way
changed in its appearance. Variolous matter kept some time,
is certainly slower in producing the disease, even where it
succeeds in the end."—*Currie's Report*, vol. i, p. 61—
Haygarth's Sketch, p. 417. According to Doctor Thomas,
" variolous and vaccine matter, by being kept for any length
of time, particularly in a warm place, is apt to undergo a decomposition by putrefaction, and then another kind of contagious matter has been produced."—P. 249.   7th. *The contagions differ in regard to the form of disease they induce.*—With
regard to the diseases they occasion, perhaps the best division
is into acute and chronic, or those attended with fever, as
small-pox, measles, scarlatina, hooping-cough, plague, yellow
and typhus fever, &c. and those which are not so accompanied,
as itch, syphilis, sibbens, yaws, elephantiasis, &c. &c. &c.
8th. *In the number of the varieties in each species of disease.*—In most, if not in all contagious diseases, there are
more than one kind ; but as the different varieties in each

have not yet been accurately fixed, we must at present con
tent ourselves by merely stating the fact.   9th. *The contagions differ from each other with regard to the organs they
affect.*—Most contagions seem to solicit expulsion by some
organ or other, and the diseases they occasion are in some
instances shorter in duration, in proportion as this expulsive
power is manifest.   Hence, where the process is active, the
creative process is shorter in duration, the system becoming
sooner exhausted.   A great proportion of the acute as well
as chronic contagions principally affect the skin.   They
differ, however, in this, that the latter are more confined to
this organ, whereas, the former affect the whole system at
the same time.   Other contagions affect the glandular system
more particularly; plague, syphilis, and mumps, are examples of this kind.   Some produce their apparent effects on
the soft parts only, others on the bones at the same time as
syphilis.   Hydrophobia seizes on the muscles of deglutition,
and infects by means of the saliva; gonorrhœa affects the mucous membrane of the urethræ ; others the brain and stomach.
10th. *The contagions differ with regard to the age, sex, and
condition of the subject to which they shew the greatest partiality.*—Hence, one age is more liable to, or susceptible of,
certain contagions than others.   11th. *In their power of repe-
tition.*—Small-pox, chicken-pox, cow-pox, hooping-cough,
measles, scarlet fever, mumps, plague, typhus and yellow
fever, are not likely to occur in the same person more than
once during life. The contagions are not the only example of
this law in the animal system.   Thus two sets of teeth only
are formed in the same person during life.   In cases where
the actions of the system so restricted, are imperfectly performed in the first instance, the same exemption from repe-
tition will not hold.   The production of ten teeth in one
jaw, will not prevent the cutting of ten teeth in the other, or
the appearance of the whole number at an after period.

     Certain idiosyncrasies existing in some individuals may
produce results different from the general rule.   Thus many

instances have occurred of persons, who, after having had two complete sets of teeth at the usual periods of life, had a third set at a very advanced age. In like manner, instances are recorded of persons being severely pitted with small-pox, who died of a second attack of that disease. The chronic contagions, viz. itch, syphilis, sibbens, yaws, elephantiasis, &c. may all be repeated in the same person. In the latter diseases the action is more local.

It is of great importance, in a practical point of view, to ascertain whether the part or constitution, or either, is susceptible of small-pox, or cow-pox, when a puncture is made, and matter applied. The following rules are given by Dr. Adams.—See *Morbid Poisons*, p. 9.

1st. If neither the part nor the constitution is susceptible, the puncture heals like the effects of any common injury.

2d. If the part only is susceptible, inflammation takes place *early*, and suppuration *soon* follows, with little or no fever.

3d. If the constitution as well as the part is susceptible, the local action takes place *more slowly*, as if interrupted by the constitutional *disposition*. As the local action advances the suppuration is preceded by the constitutional action, and the disease becomes general. The host of darning-needle practitioners, who believe the whole art of inoculation and vaccination, to consist in making the puncture, should be made aware of the skill and discrimination such matters require, and even medical men should in all cases recollect (which many of them do not), that it is the constitutional action *fully and completely exerted*, which can alone give any hopes of security.

Such are the most remarkable differences observable amongst the contagions. They differ likewise in their power of infection, in other words, in strength and certainty of action; also, in the time they remain latent in the system. These last will be treated of in another place.

We before noticed a distinction which some writers have

attempted to make amongst them, viz. infections and contagions, according to the meaning of the terms given by Rush. Professor Hosack has answered this theory successfully. According to his method, we shall suppose *A.* to be ill of typhus fever, a disease well known to be attended with a peculiar train of symptoms; he is in a small confined apartment, his person is neglected, the air around him is rendered impure and offensive. Under these circumstances *B.* visits him, and a few days after is also taken sick with the *same disease,* attended in all respects with the same dangerous symptoms which mark the disorder of *A.* Dr. Rush, and those who adopt the doctrine of *infection,* as opposed to *contagion,* consider the disease of *B.* to proceed *from the impurities of the air* of the chamber, and not any thing *peculiar* emanating or secreted from the body of *A.* But as we may *without hazard* visit an equally filthy chamber where *C.* is confined with a broken limb, we therefore ascribe the disease of *B.* to something more than the *impure air* of the chamber of *A.* We ascribe it to a peculiar *virus* generated in his system by the disease under which he labours, and communicated by his effluvia to the surrounding atmosphere, rendering it thus capable of producing the same disease in those who may be exposed to its influence.—*(On Contagion).*

The power of the atmosphere in increasing and diminishing contagious diseases of the febrile kind does not seem to be quite understood. From our own observations made in different climates, we are disposed to think that cold, by diminishing fever, may frequently diminish, or even destroy the creative process; but that the very same degree of cold acts injuriously in some instances by condensing the atmosphere, and thus enabling it to suspend the contagion already formed. On the other hand, we think that heat, by increasing fever, is favourable to the generative power, but by rarefying the atmosphere, and enforcing cleanliness and ventilation, it is unfavourable to the contagion, excepting in places where it is present in a very concentrated form. According to this theory, small-pox spreads with greater difficulty in Britain during Winter from two causes: 1st. The cold lessens the fever—2nd. It hinders or suspends the action of the agent by freezing that matter which, even in Summer, exists partly in a palpable fluid form. Did small-pox contagion exist only in a subtle, invisible and impalpable form, like that of typhus, the cold of Winter would have proved unfavorable to its spreading in one way, but favorable in another. Again, the contagion of plague, which probably exists in a medium state between the gross matter of small-pox and the subtle virus of typhus, is destroyed or injured either by great heat, or by great cold. Upon the whole, we are inclined to believe that temperature acts chiefly in the manner we have described, and not so much by any specific power that heat or cold exerts on the contagions themselves. The influence of temperature in generating contagion is best exemplified in hydrophobia.

Effects of Crowding, Filth, &c.

The rise and progress of most of the great epidemics on record, have been closely connected with some extraordinary condition of mankind.

In the sacred volume there are these words :—" Thus saith the Lord; him that is in the *open field* will I give to the beasts to be devoured, and they that be *in the forts and the cities shall die of the pestilence.*" In the 25th chapter of Jeremiah, where the prophet foretels the siege of Jerusalem, it is said, " I will smite the inhabitants of this city, both men and beasts, they shall die with great pestilence. *He that abideth in this city,* shall die by the sword, by the famine, and by the pestilence ; but he that *goeth out,* falleth to the Chaldeans that besiege you, *he shall live,* and his life shall be to him as a prey."

A pestilential disease raged in Greece and neighbouring countries of Asia, after the destruction of Troy; and Herodotus attributes it to the miseries occasioned by the Trojan war.

The famous plague of Athens began in the second year of the Peloponnesian war, which ravaged Greece for twenty-seven years. According to Thucydides, Archidamus, with an army of 60,000 men, laid waste the beautiful plains of Attica, and compelled the inhabitants to seek refuge within the walls of their crowded and populous city. "The Athenians," says Diodorus Siculus, in lib. xii, " not daring to meet their enemies, the Peloponnesians, in open battle in the plains, remained cooped up within their walls, and caused pestilential effluvia, for great numbers of people congregating in the city, very readily *generated the disease* by breathing a corrupted air;" and Plutarch tells us, " that Pericles was accused of giving greater violence to the pestilence, by involving his country in this destructive war, and by keeping the people cooped up like herds of cattle, *to be infected with contagion from one another.*"—(Vide *Vita Pericles*). " Crowds of people were crammed into the turrets of the walls, or wherever they could find a vacant corner. Even the Pelasgie, a hitherto vacant spot of ground below the citadel, the occupation of which was contrary to the express prohibition of the Pythian Oracle, they were constrained by necessity to turn into a dwelling-place. The people that had come in from the country had no houses, but dwelt all the Summer in stifling booths, where there was scarce room to breathe." *The physicians and all who attended the sick, were cut off by the contagion.*—Vide *Thucydides.*

The influx of inhabitants is stated, by a late writer, to have been from 50 to 400,000. Thucydides gives a melancholy account of the conduct of the people during the rage of this pestilence. " Men," he says, " grew careless both of holy and profane things alike. Neither the fear of God nor laws of man awed any one; men thought they held their lives but by the day; what any man knew to be delightful and profitable pleasure, that was made both profitable and honourable. Hence, every species of pillage and vice went on without restraint, as no one believed his life would last till he received punishment for his crimes. The mortality was without all form; dying men lay tumbling over one another in the streets, and even the temples where they dwelt in tents, were all full of the dead that had died within them."

Dionysius, the Halicarnassian historian, gives accounts of pestilential fevers in different parts of his Roman History, and in these he makes direct allusion to contagion. In the 451st year before the Christian æra, and about 300 after the building of Rome, " the most pestilential disease ever remembered brought destruction on the city, by which almost all those affording assistance were cut off; nearly one-half of the other citizens were destroyed. Neither were the physicians able to attend the sick, nor the friends nor domestics to administer the necessaries, for they who willingly attended others, by touching their diseased bodies or dwelling with them, were seized with the same malady."—*Dionysii Halicarnassensis Historia, Oxoniæ,* 1704, *p.* 645.

This historian has given a lively and pathetic description of the deplorable condition of the city during the ravages caused by the disease. He says, " the stench from the unburied dead bodies, which were cast into the sewers or the high-ways, and into the river, and again thrown by the tide on its banks, contributed to maintain the disease by spreading the infection ; for such was the desolation, that whole houses were deprived of their inhabitants by death. The contagion was carried into the country, where numbers perished, and the Æqui, Volsci and Sabines, enemies of Rome, desirous of taking advantage of the distresses of the city, by invading it, received the infection, and carried destruction into their own dwellings."

In Diodorus's history, there are also accounts of pestilential diseases happening in different parts of the world, but particularly *among multitudes of people collected for the purposes of war.* The contagious pestilence which broke out at Carthage, at the time it was invaded by Dionysius, the tyrant of Syracuse, is particularly described by him, and the description given, has a strong resemblance to that of other historians, but particularly to the one given above of the plague of Rome. " As the mortality," says Diodorus, "caused by the disease was great, and as the attendants on the sick were cut off by it, no one dared to approach the infected :" and again he adds, " for all took the disease who had close communication with the sick, so that wretched indeed was the condition of those who were diseased, every one being unwilling to visit ; for not only they who were not bound by any tie of relationship deserted the sick, but near brothers and friends were compelled to neglect their nearest relations on account of the dread of contagion." The pestilential fever which broke out in Rome about the year 389, A. U. C. made its appearance under similar circumstances.

Livy states that, " not only the inhabitants of the country but even the cattle *were crowded into the city,* in order to find shelter from the ravages of the enemy, and both men and cattle were affected with equal malignity. Such a confused collection of animals of every kind affected the citizens by the unusual stench, while the country people, crowded in narrow apartments, suffered no less from the heat, the want of rest, and their attendance on each other. Besides, even contact served to propagate the infection." The words of Livy are "Grave tempus et forte annus pestilens erat urbi agrisque, nec hominibus magis, quam pecori ; et auxere vim morbi, terrore populationis pecoribus agrestibusque in urbem acceptis. Ea conluvio mixtorum omnis generis animantium et odore insolito urbanos, et agrestem, confertum in arta tecta æstu ac vigiliis angebat, ministeriaque in vicem ac contagio ipsa vulgabant morbos."—*Livy,* lib. iii. c. vi. p. 47.

Dionysius of Halicarnassus, notices similar facts in lib. x. and Orosius, in his account of the same fever, observes (lib. ii.)

—Many of the patricians were victims, but it was most fatal to the poor. Livy makes a similar observation, that many illustrious persons died, but that among those of inferior rank, the virulence of the disorder spread its ravages wide.

A great mortality took place among the troops at the siege of Syracuse by Marcellus, a siege rendered memorable by the death of Archimedes. It raged among those of both sides, but more particularly among the Carthagenians, who all perished with their generals, Hippocrates and Homilis. According to Livy, who gives an account of this disease, " the pestilence broke out in both armies, which directed their minds from the concerns of war, for *it was in Autumn, and in a situation naturally unhealthy.* The heat, which was more *without* the city than *within,* affected almost every person in both the camps ; but first, persons sickened and died by means of the unwholesomeness of the place ; afterwards, the disease *spread by infection,* so that those who were seized were neglected or abandoned, and died, *or their attendants contracted the same disease."* " Daily burials and deaths were before their eyes, and day and night their ears were assailed with lamentations. At length the survivors became hardened ; they neither grieved at the death of others, nor took pains to bury the dead, and the bodies of the deceased lay scattered along the streets in sight of those who were expecting the same fate. The dead infected the sick, and the sick those in health with terror and pestiferous stench, and some, preferring death by the sword, rushed on the ports of the enemy." But the disease was much more severe to the Carthagenians than to the Romans, who, in this long siege, had become accustomed to the air and water. The Sicilian troops, on the first breaking out of the disease, abandoned their allies, and returned to their houses. The Carthagenians, who had no means of shelter, all perished. Many, however, of the Roman army died of the disease. The words of Livy are—" Accessit et pestilentia, commune malum, quod facile utrorumque animos averteret a belli consiliis: *nam tempore autumni, et locis natura gravibus,* multo tamen magis *extra* urbem, quam *in* urbe, intoleranda vis æstus per utraque castra omnium ferme corpora movit. Et primo temporis ac loci vitio et ægri erant, et moriebantur: postea curatio ipsa *et contactus ægrorum vulgabat morbos:* ut aut neglecti desertique, qui incidissent, morerentur, aut adsidentes curantesque eadem vi morbi repletos secum traherent."—*Lib.* xxv. cap. 26.

In the few extracts from ancient history given above, we have it clearly demonstrated how much disease depends on human actions, and how intimately contagion is connected with certain states of society, particularly congregations of men collected and crowded together for the purposes of war. That the ancients attributed these pestilential diseases to their true causes is indisputable; for, besides the facts quoted from them, several historians, philosophers, physicians, and poets, make direct allusion to contagion. Those who are fond of pursuing this subject may consult the works of Aristotle,* Galen,† Aretæus, Ammianus Marcellinus,‡ Virgil,§ Lucretius,‖ Ovid,¶ Lucan and Sillus Italicus.

The more modern history of pestilential diseases furnishes one continued train of the same remarkable facts. In a work however, of this kind, it is not possible to give many such accounts, nor is it necessary, since every one moderately acquainted with history must know them.

The description of London before and after the great fire of 1666, will suffice to give a pretty correct notion of the state of the other great cities of Europe about the same period. " The streets were narrow, crowded, and many of them unpaved: the houses were built of wood, and lofty; they were dark, irregular, and ill-constructed, with each story hanging over the one below, so as almost to meet at top and thereby preclude as much as possible all access to a pure air;

---

* Problem 8th, Section 7th.   † Lib. i. Cap. iii. de Febribus.
‡ Lib. xiv. Cap. vi.   § Eclogue 1st, and Georgics, Lib. iii.
‖ De Rerum Natura.   ¶ Metamor. Lib. vii.

they were besides furnished with enormous signs, which, by
hanging into the middle of the street, contributed not a little
to prevent all ventilation below. The sewers at the same
time were in a very neglected state, and the drains all ran
above ground : add to which, the metropolis, which now
enjoys such a plentiful supply of water, had been but scantily
supplied with water."

" In 1389, the streets of London were so abused with
common lay-stalls, to the great annoyance of the citizens,
that a proclamation was made throughout the city, by authority of Parliament—' That no person whatever should presume
' to lay any dung, guts, garbage, offals, or any other ordure,
' in any street, ditch, river, &c. upon penalty of twenty pounds,
' to be recovered by an information in Chancery.' "—Vide
*Maitland's History, and Heberden on the Increase and
Decrease of Diseases.* The internal arrangements of the
houses in London, &c. corresponded with the description of
the streets. Erasmus, in a letter to Franciscus, physician to
Cardinal Wolsey, ascribes the sweating sickness and the
plague itself to the slovenly habits of the people, both without
and within doors. " The floors," he says, " are commonly of
clay strewed with rushes, which are occasionally renewed,
but underneath lies unmolested an ancient collection of beer,
grease, fragments of filth, spittle, the excrements of dogs
and cats, and every thing that is nasty."—*History of
England.*

Holingshed, who lived in the reign of Queen Elizabeth,
speaking of the increase of luxury, says, " there are old men
yet dwelling in the village where I remain, who have noted
three things to be marvellously altered in England within
their own remembrance. One is the number of chimneys
lately erected ; whereas, in their young days, there were not
above *two or three, if so many,* in most uplandish towns of
the realm—(the religious houses and manor places of their
lords always excepted, and peradventure some great personage), but each made his fire against a reredosse in the hall,

where he dined and dressed his meat. The second is the great amendment in lodging ; for said they, our fathers, and we ourselves, have lain full oft on straw-pallets, covered only with a sheet, under coverlets made of dogswaine, hop-harlots, (I use their own terms), and a good round log under their head for a bolster."* The same author and Maitland may be consulted for further information. Hume remarks, that we may form a notion of the mean way of living in the 16th cencentury, from one circumstance : a man of no less rank than the Comptroller to Edward the Sixth's household, paid only thirty shillings a year for a house in Channel Row, yet labour and provisions, and consequently houses, were only about a third below the present price."—*History of England.* Hentzner, speaking of the presence-chamber at Greenwich Palace, in the time of Queen Elizabeth, observes—that " the floor after the English fashion was strewed with hay." " In what a comparative state of filth," says Bateman, " if a degree of comparison *lower than this can be conceived,* must the poor have lived in those times—the poor who now occupy in separate apartments the very houses in the courts and alleys in London, which were formerly inhabited by the rich, even by the Comptroller of the King's household."—*Reports, p.* 17.

The history of disease during this period, furnishes a train of facts which ought never to be forgotten.

In the 14th, 15th, and 16th centuries, there scarcely passed ten years without a considerable plague. The greatest plague years of the 17th century, were 1603, 1625, 1636, 1665, in which the mortality by plague alone is reported to be respectively 36,000, 35,000, 10,000, and 68,000. By referring to these numbers it will be seen, that plague followed the law of a true contagion, in raging to a considerable extent only at distant periods, thus always affording time for a new and susceptible race to spring up. That the same individuals

---

* Hume, vol. iv. p. 315.

were not liable to the disease twice likewise appears from this, that the longer the interval between two epidemic visits, the greater was the mortality, and *vice versa.* Thus, after the shortest interval, viz. between the years 1625 and 1636, eleven years, the mortality by plague was only 10,000; whereas, after the longest interval, viz. between 1636 and 1665, 68,000 died of it; and Lord Clarendon, in the history of his own life, says, " many who could compute very well, concluded there were double that number." We are told by Hodges, that, in 1665, " the city was unusually full of people, for the wars being over, the armies disbanded, and the Royal Family and Monarchy restored, they had flocked to London to settle in business"—so that we are furnished with another reason why the mortality was so much greater in the latter year, there having been, according to some accounts, an influx of more than a hundred thousand strangers. But London was by no means free from plague at other periods. In 1604, 900 died of plague; in 1605, 400; in 1606, 2,000; in 1607, 2,000; in 1608, 2,000; in 1609, 4,000; in 1610, 1,800; and from 1640 to 1648, the number was every year above 1,000. Heberden is of opinion, that some years might have passed without any deaths from plague; but he quotes Maitland, who, in his History of London, declares, that for five and twenty years before the fire of 1666, the city had never been free from the disease; another convincing proof that plague (to use the words of Hodges before quoted), continually wants *something* to keep it up. The contagion, though never absent for twenty-five years, a quarter of a century, was yet unable to extend itself, till that *something*, in the shape of a mass of human beings, or a crowd of susceptible strangers, arrived. It was then the dreadful mortality began, as it had always done before, among the poor. L'Estrange remarks, that the plagues of 1625 and 1636, began in Whitechapel; in 1666, it began in St. Giles, where the principal mortality took place. Both Hodges and the author of the history of that plague, agree in stating, it was so much con-

fined to the poor that it got the name of " the poor's plague ;"
30 or 40,000 of its victims were believed to be servants out
of place, p. 199. In other words, the strangers and others
"seeking for business." We have here a very remarkable
and humiliating proof of the evil tendency of false theory,
in blinding us to the real causes of human misery, namely,
human misrule. The philosopher, the physician, the peer,
and the pauper, seem all to have been alike ignorant of contagion, the real cause of disease. While engaged with his
telescope and horoscope, the weather-wiseman had no time
to contemplate sublunary objects, and the study of the constitutions of the atmosphere was thought to be of more consequence by the physician, than a knowledge of the construction of towns and dwellings, or of the human constitution.
As to the poor, "they were," says the author of the history,
" the most venturous and fearless, and went about with *a
sort of brutal courage, as it was founded neither on religion
nor prudence.*" Upon the whole, less seems to have been
known of the nature of contagion and of the evils arising
from human effluvia in a close and crowded state of society,
in the days of Sydenham, Hodges, Mead, and Short, than in
the time of Thucydides, and the other ancient historians
before quoted.

In September, 1666, while the plague was yet raging, happened the memorable fire of London. It raged for several
days together, till it had consumed every thing from the
Tower to Temple Bar. This, which was at first looked upon
as a scourge from heaven, has since proved a most gracious
blessing.

Great pains were taken, and much encouragement given
by the King, to obtain proper plans for building the city : the
streets were widened, drains and cesspools made, the lay-
stalls and huge signs removed, &c. ; orders were issued to
sweep and cleanse the streets, lanes, and common passages,
"from dung, soil, filth and dirt ;" all persons were forbid to
lay in the streets any dogs, cats, inwards of beasts, cleaves of

beasts, feet, bones, horns, dregs, or dross of ale or beer, or any noisome thing, upon pain of ten shillings for every offence. It was ordered also that no man shall feed any kine, goats, hogs, or poultry, in the open streets; that no man cast into ditches, or sewers, grates, or gullets of the city, any manner of carrion, stinking flesh, rotten oranges, or onions, rubbish, dung, &c. &c.; that no man shall make, or continue any widraughts, seat or seats for houses of easement over, or drains into any common sewers, and other regulations were enforced to the same effect.—*Maitland's History*. So that in a few years the new town rose like a phœnix from the fire, with increased vigour and beauty. Nor did the benefit end here, for it produced in the country a spirit of improvement, which had till then been unknown, but which has never since ceased to exert itself.—*Heberden, p.* 76-7.

A corresponding change took place in the diseases, and particularly of plague. In 1665, 68,000 died of it; in 1666, the year of the fire, 4,998; in the year following 35, and the year after that 14; since which time the number has never exceeded *five;* and the last year it is mentioned in the bills is 1679, notwithstanding the population and the trade of London have been so rapidly increasing since that time. The change in other diseases was not less wonderful. In 1624, the mortality from other diseases was 12,199; in 1625, 18,848; in 1626, 7,400; in 1635, 10,051; in 1636, 12,958; in 1637, 8,641; in 1664, 18,291; in 1665, the year of the great plague, 28,710; in 1666, the year of the fire, 10,840. Remittents, intermittents, dysentery, and other bowel complaints, rickets, scurvy, &c., were the prevailing diseases.

Even during the 18th century, the metropolis was a great vortex, in which several thousands of emigrants from the country annually perished. The following is the average excess of the deaths above the births in each year, during the first, second, fourth, and last ten years of the century. First ten years or decade, the average excess of deaths above the births each year was 5,788 ; the annual average of the excess in the second decade, was 6,798 ; in the fourth, 9,662 ; but in the last ten years of the century it was only 926.

In the first decade of the present century the thing is reversed, for, from the year 1801 till 1810, both inclusive, the annual average in favour of the births is 1,412; and in the seven subsequent years, that is up to 1818, the births have exceeded the deaths by an annual average of 2,952. The decrease of deaths from bowel complaints is very remarkable. In the first decade of the 18th century, the annual average of deaths from bowel complaints is 1,070 ; second decade, 770 ; third, 700 ; fourth, 350 ; fifth, 150 ; sixth, 110 ; seventh, 80 ; eighth, 70 ; ninth, 40 ; and in the tenth decade, *viz.*, from 1790 to 1800, the annual average of deaths from bowel complaints is only 20. During the 18th century, when the whole deaths in London amounted to about 21,000 yearly, the following is the annual average of deaths, from evil, in a decade, at the beginning, middle, and end of it:—beginning, 70 ; middle, 15 ; end, 8—rickets, beginning, 380; middle, 11 ; end, 1.

It may be interesting to stop here, and enquire why Sydenham and his cotemporaries so strangely overlooked contagion in plague, and even small-pox, seeing that the power of the former to propagate itself under similar circumstances, had been directly alluded to by so many authors before their time. Dr. Adams, has given perhaps the best explanation that can be given of this fact. He observes, " In these temperate regions, and in that comparatively easy state in which the majority exist even in this overgrown metropolis, diseases assume a milder aspect ; but if we trace them in countries nearer the sun, in camps, or in the writings of Sydenham, during whose practice London was little better than a garrison, and in some respects worse, we find some one disease constantly prevailing and succeeding another in proportion to the force of each; sometimes determined by the seasons varying with them, alternating with infection, and superseding or giving way to different contagions. Under such circumstances, it would not be easy to make a distinction between endemics, epidemics, infections, and contagions. All will appear to owe their origin to one common cause, all will seem to commence in a similar manner, and such will be the transition from one to the other, that it will be difficult to fix the exact limits of each."—*On Morbid Poisons, p.* 323. It is from the same reasons that medical men who have only seen contagious diseases in camps, garrisons, or in ships, in hot climates, where the high temperature, marsh and human effluvia, all conspire in giving something of a common character to very different diseases, so frequently overlook the effects of contagion altogether. The difficulty of tracing it in a crowded population, the many ways in which it is often spread without apparent communication with the sick, the escape of others actually exposed, owing to the better ventilation in such climates, the nonsusceptibility of persons to a second attack, or from the previous occupation of their systems with other diseases, are all circumstances tending to give a deceptive feature to diseases known to be contagious. Medical men, whose practice has been chiefly confined to the army and navy in hot climates, frequently fall into the very error that Sydenham committed, in attributing contagious diseases to an endemic origin. Thus, some of them contend that the intermittent, remittent, and continued fevers of such climates, are only different forms of the same disease, and arise from the same cause, marsh poison, in a different degree of concentration or force. Sydenham, describes the intermittent and continued fevers of 1661, as beginning with the same symptoms, and as if originating in similar causes ; but he says, " the intermittent constitution *ceased with the Autumn,* when the continued fever was uninterrupted in its course ; in other words, the continued or worst form, according to the endemic theory, began to manifest itself when its supposed cause, marsh effluvia, ceased to operate, but became vigorous and uninterrupted in its course when human effluvia became

more concentrated and more powerful. The modern sup-
porters of endemic or natural causes commit blunders equally
conspicuous. For instance, who could frame an apology for
Dr. Adams's error, in conceiving a thing so absurd and pre-
posterous as a stratum of pestiferous air, extending from
China to Charing Cross, that air being impregnated with an
endemic poison, or one arising from human bodies."—*Morb.
Pois. p.* 356.

The plague was not confined to London, but extended to
Scotland and different parts of the island; but we know of
no city where births and burials have been so regularly re-
gistered as in the metropolis. Life and death are not yet
counted matters of sufficient importance in Scotland to deserve being regularly recorded. With the exception of crimi-
nals who make their exit on a scaffold, the great majority
are allowed to come in and go out of the world the best way
they can; and, as hanging has never been endemic, epidemic,
or contagious in this part of the empire, the criminal cal-
lendar does not fall under our notice. Bessy Bell and Mary
Gray, the subjects of the celebrated Scotch song, bearing the
same title, are said to have died of the plague in the year of
the great fire of London. The common tradition is, that the
father of the former was Laird of Kinnaird, in the neighbourhood of Lyndock, and the father of the latter Laird of Lyndock—that these two young ladies were both very handsome, and a most intimate friendship subsisted between them;
that, while Miss Bell was on a visit to Miss Gray, the plague
broke out in the year 1666. In order to avoid which, they
built themselves a bower, about three-quarters of a mile west
from Lyndock-house, in a very retired and romantic place,
called Burn-bræ, on the side of Branchie-burn, where they
lived for some time, but the plague raging with great fury,
they caught the infection, it is said from a young gentleman
who was in love with both, and here they died. The burial-
place lies about half a mile west from the present house of
Lyndock.—Vide *Muses Thronodie, p.* 19—*Perth,* 1774.

It appears from the following extracts from the ancient records of the Burgh of Linlithgow, that strong measures were enforced at a very early period with a view of preventing the spreading of the contagion of plague. These extracts were in the hand-writing of the late Sir Alexander Seaton, who was many years Provost (Mayor) of the town, and as they are, without doubt, copies verbatim from the books, and faithfully copied by ourselves, their authenticity may be depended upon. We consider them creditable to that very respectable Burgh, considering the state of science at the time the facts were recorded.

4th Dec. 1625.—Plague in Edinburgh; dykes repaired; watched night and day; no admittance without order of Bailie (Magistrate). *13th January,* 1625, (nearly a year before) —Inhabitants discharged (forbid) from harbouring any suspected of witchcraft, sorcery, or under-bruit. *11th September,* 1637—The plague in Holland; precautions adopted and recommended; eight men watch; yard dykes mended. *18th April,* 1645—Plague in Edinburgh and country around, and at Boness; the watch enforced. *14th July,* 1645—The inhabitants discharged (forbid) to go to Edinburgh; plague increasing; parliament at Stirling. *18th July,* 1645—Magdalen fair discharged on account of plague; strong watch at the ports. *27th November,* 1645—Request from Provost of Edinburgh to provide accommodation at Linlithgow, during the plague, to the college and students; the Counsel assign them the Kirk to be divided by themselves. *17th October,* 1648—Precautions still used against the plague and pestilence, particularly forbidding visiting of the sick. *July* 2, 1650—The plague not altogether subsided. *January* 20, 1660—Annual list of burials by the officers, and of baptisms by session clerk, layed in counsel amrie.

Arnot gives, in his History of Edinburgh, the copy of an order from the Privy Counsel of Edinburgh, which equally banished to Inchkeith, a desolate island in the Firth of Forth, those who were affected with the venereal disease, and those who undertook to cure it. It appears from the extracts above referred to, that the inhabitants of Linlithgow were treated with much greater sympathy by their town council; for those labouring under this malady were not only allowed the benefit of the healing art, but were actually cured at the Burgh expense. Precautions were taken against the spreading of venereal disease at a still earlier period. There is a fragment of an Act of Parliament preserved of the time of Henry II. (A.D. 1162), for regulating the Stews, in which it is ordained, among other things, "that no stew-holder shall keep a woman who has the perilous infirmity of burning."—*Stow's Survey*, c. ii. p. 7.

The plague of 1665, " which raged in most parts of the kingdom, never visited any person in Oxford, *although the terms were there kept, and the court and both houses of parliament did there reside.*" Dr. Plott, from whose History of Oxfordshire, this fact is taken, attributes the exemption of Oxford, to the clean, open, and better-ventilated streets, and to the care of the magistrates and Richard Fox, bishop of Winchester, at a very early period, *viz.* 1517, to drain the town. Besides, Oxford being then the seat of the court and both houses of parliament, must have been chiefly occupied by the higher ranks of people, among whom the disease was so little felt that, Lord Clarendon affirms, " when he and other persons of condition who had fled from the plague, returned to London, they hardly missed one of their friends and acquaintances, the mortality having been confined almost entirely to the lowest order of people."—The same observation has been made everywhere.

The plague of Dantzic, in 1709, first appeared in a low dirty part of the city.—*Webster.* At Alet, in 1720, scarcely more than one or two of the whole number of persons infected by the plague was above the lowest class.—See *Sauvage's Nos. Method.* This was also the case at Copenhagen, in 1711; for, according to Gottwald, the plague was

M

generally most fatal to the meanest sort. Out of a population of about 60,000 when it began, 25,000 died; yet, among
all these, scarcely one person of note. The reason assigned
for the poor being the principal victims, were their filthiness
and close manner of living, three or four families being confined to a single room.—*Short*, vol. ii. p. 7. The plague of
Marseilles, in 1720, cut off 60,000 of its inhabitants. It
began in the Rue de le Scalle, a place noted for the sordid
filth, crowded state, and wretchedness of the poor inhabitants. Bertrand, in his " Relation Historique," says that,
at first, none fell victims to it but children and poor people.
At length the disease got into the Hôtel Dieu, destroying
the nurses, physicians, surgeons, apothecaries, confessors,
and all fhe attendants on the sick, with the whole of the poor
of the hospital, including above three hundred foundlings.
The whole city at last became more or less one infirmary.—
See *Bertrands, City Remembrancer*, Sec. 111—*Ingram on
Plague, &c.* At Rensburgh, in Holstein, in 1764, it broke
out in crowded situations, inhabited by the lower classes
(Heberden); also at Cronstadt, as stated by Chenot in his
history. In the plague of Moscow, which happened in 1771,
out of a population of about 150,000, 80,000 died; and
Mertins, who practised there at the time, and who has
written an account of the epidemic, says, " I only knew of
three noblemen who were attacked by the disease, very few
respectable tradesmen, and only three hundred strangers of
the lowest condition. All the rest were Russians of the inferior class." Thus, we see the poor are the chief sufferers
from plague. Dr. Heberden, thinks this is true universally;
Mertins asserts, that it has usually happened; and even
Mead says, " it has hardly ever been known that the disease
did not first appear among the lower order."—*Mead's Works,*
p. 165.

The exact same thing holds good in typhus fever; and
who does not know that this scourge almost always exists,

EFFECTS OF CROWDING, FILTH, ETC.

more or less, in the narrow, crowded and filthy parts of all our great towns, when the cleaner and better-aired quarters of them are seldom visited.

Dr. Willan, when speaking of applications to charitable institutions for relief, observes, "The good effects of all these applications are often superseded by the miserable accommodations of the poor, with respect to bedding, and by a total neglect of ventilation in their narrow, crowded dwellings. It will scarcely appear credible, though it is precisely true, that persons of the lowest class do not put clean sheets on their beds three times a year ; that, even where no sheets are used, they never wash or scour their blankets and coverlets, nor renew them till they are no longer tenable; that curtains, if unfortunately there should be any, are never cleaned, but suffered to continue in the same state till they drop to pieces ; lastly, that from three to eight individuals of different ages often sleep in the same bed, there being in general but one room and one bed for each family. To the above circumstances may be added, that the room occupied is either a deep cellar almost inaccessible to the light and admitting of no change of air, or a garret, with a low roof and small windows, the passage to which is close, kept dark in order to lessen the window-tax, and filled not only with bad air, but with putrid, excremental or other abominable effluvia from a vault at the bottom of the staircase. Washing of linen or some other disagreeable business is carried on, while infants are left dosing, and children more advanced kept at play whole days in the tainted bed ; some unsavoury victuals are from time to time cooked; in many instances idleness, in others the cumbrous furniture or utensils of trade with which the apartments are clogged, prevent the salutary operations of the broom and whitewashing brush, and favour the accumulation of a heterogeneous fermenting filth. From all these causes combined, there is necessarily produced a complication of fetor, to describe which, would be as vain an attempt as for those to conceive who have always been accustomed to neat and comfortable dwellings." — Vide *Willan's Reports, p.* 257.

The above description of the habitations of the poor in London, Westminster, &c., is in conformity with that given by a still later writer on the diseases of the metropolis. Dr. Clutterbuck, in a book published on the Epidemic Fever of 1816, gives this picture of some parts of modern London :— " The houses they occupy (the poor) are often large, and every room has its family, from the cellar to the garret ; thirty or forty individuals are thus often collected together under the same roof. The different apartments must be approached by a common staircase, which is rarely washed or cleaned ; there are often no doors or openings of any kind backwards, and the privies are not unfrequently within the walls, and emit a loathsome stench that is diffused over the whole house ; the houses are generally situated in long and narrow alleys, with lofty buildings on each side, or in a small confined court which has but a single opening, and that perhaps a low gateway. Such a court is, in fact, little other than a well. These places are at the same time the receptacles of all kinds of filth, which is only removed by the scavenger at distant and uncertain intervals, and always so imperfectly as to leave the place highly offensive and disgusting."—Pp. 44-5.

No one can read these accounts of parts of modern London, which must have been portions of the new town that rose like a phœnix in the midst of the great fire in 1666, without being convinced that such habitations are the very hot-beds of contagion. We are at the same time induced to ask the question—how the plague disappeared while such abodes continued ?

The population of London must have continued very low for many years after the fire, if we can judge from that of both England and Wales. Mr. Rickman, in a computation founded on the return of baptisms, as stated in the abstract of parish registers, makes the population of 1700 amount to 5,475,000; that of 1750, to 6,467,000 ; that of 1770, to

7,428,000. The first actual enumeration was in 1801, which gave to England and Wales, 9,168,000; the census of 1811 made it 10,488,000; that of 1821, gives 11,977,668; and the census of 1831, 13,977,688; so that the increase between 1811 and 1821, was 1,827,048, a number more than equal to the whole population of England (exclusive of Wales) at the Norman conquest, and probably greater than what it was three hundred years afterwards. It is stated in the parliamentary reports, that the annual mortality of London in 1700 was 1 in 25; in 1750, 1 in 21; in 1801, and the four preceding years, 1 in 35; in 1810, 1 in 38. It further appears, that the census of 1801, makes the mortality of England and Wales 1 in 44·8 of the year in which it was taken; that of 1811, makes the average mortality 1 in 48·7.

The population of Ireland has advanced in a most surprising manner likewise. Sir William Petty, in his Political Anatomy of Ireland, p. 17, estimates it at 1,100,000 in 1672. It has advanced to about seven millions in 150 years.

It would be of great importance could the annual deaths from fever in London be accurately ascertained. Dr. Stanger computed the number of fever cases in London yearly, at 40,000.—*On Contagion, p.* 39.—Willan in his Reports, p. 332, states the annual average of deaths from infectious fever, within the bills of mortality, during the last century, at 3,188; in all, 318,800.

In Liverpool, at a period when the population did not exceed 63,000, above 3,000 patients labouring under contagious fever, were annually admitted to the benefits of the dispensary. Above 7,000 persons live in cellars under ground, and 9,000 in back-houses, which have an imperfect ventilation; and in the cellars and back-houses contagion is constantly present. The prevalence of contagious fever will account for the enormous poor-rate which, in this town, amounted in the year 1801 to £2,800.—Vide *Clark's Papers.* The mortality of Liverpool was 1 in 34, on an average of ten years; and 1 in 30, in the year 1811. Manchester, when it was the second town in England in point of population, was healthier than the rest of Lancashire. The mortality there, on an average of ten years, was 1 in 58; and in the year 1811, 1 in 74. In the year 1757, according to the late Dr. Perceval, the annual mortality of Manchester, was 1 in 25·7; and in 1770, 1 in 28, although at the former period, the population was not quite one-fourth; and at the latter period not one half of its present amount.—Vide *Perceval Works.* Dr. Perceval at this time introduced some enlightened measures of medical police, which have since been continued by Dr. Ferriar.

Between the years 1811 and 1822, the city of Edinburgh and town of Leith had increased in population 32,000, a number equal to its whole population in 1752, so that they increased one hundred thousand in sixty years. In 1752, when the population of Edinburgh and Canongate was some hundreds more than 32,000 and each family was believed to contain about five persons, the mortality was 1 in 30.—Vide *Edin. Med. Essays and Observations,* 1752, vol. i. The high and exposed situation of Edinburgh must always render it healthier in proportion than some other large cities—thus a free ventilation in the dwellings of the poor will frequently prevent the bad consequences arising from filth and crowding. Dr. Macculloch, in his account of the Hebrides, states, that " while the inhabitants had no shelter but huts of the most simple construction, which afforded free ingress and egress to the air, *they were not subject to fevers;* but when, through the good intentions of the proprietors, commodious and comfortable habitations were provided, but which afforded recesses for stagnating air and impurities, which they wanted the taste and cleanliness to correct, *then febrile infection was generated.*" This may be one reason why the Russians, although in many respects a filthy people, yet remain comparatively free from contagious diseases. The coldness of the climate and the universal practice of bathing themselves, will undoubtedly contribute to their health. The Russian

bills of mortality for the year 1819, give the following proofs
of longevity in the male sex:—there were 18,741 above 80 ;
5,754 above 90 ; 1,094 above 100 ; 324 above 105 ; 179
above 110 ; 90 above 115 ; 56 above 120 ; 23 above 125 ;
13 above 130 ; and two, the extraordinary age of between
140 and 150. Personal cleanliness, in a country so cold as
Russia, will cover a multitude of sins. Dr. Clark, in his
systematic growlings against those people, has scarcely done
them justice in this respect. No one can doubt that the
practice of bathing and washing the surface of the body is so
general in Russia as to be almost universal. On the other
hand, it is comparatively rare in England ; for even the better
classes of people neglect it to a degree that is scarcely credible. Lest therefore, we should not be believed, we quote
Dr. Parr, who says, in his London Medical Dictionary, art.
Coopertio, "Those who would think themselves injured if
they did not change their linen daily, will often not change
their flannel for months ;" he might have added, those who
do change both linen and flannel regularly, do not wash the
surface of their bodies for years. Amongst the many springs
and fountains dedicated to different saints, we have not been
able to find out one bearing the name of St. George—we
leave St. Andrew out of the question. Soap was not made
in London till 1554 ; a coarse kind was manufactured at
Bristol before that period.—*Anderson's History of Commerce
—Howel's Letters.* Yet, if we may judge from the writings
of some medical authors of note, it was not used as a means
of bodily cleanliness till a much later date. Diemerbroeck,
who wrote on the plague of Nimeguen in 1686, says, "he
saw three persons attacked with fever, occasioned by the
smell of soap that had been used in washing their linen ; and
Van Swieten, who lived about a century later, reprobates the
use of it. The consumption of soap has, however, increased
surprisingly since. From a speech of Lord Liverpool, in the
House of Commons, it appears that, on the average of the
years 1787 and 1788, it was 292,006,440 pounds, being about

twenty-two pounds yearly for every individual then in England, Ireland, and Scotland; but on the average of years
from 1816 to 1821, it amounted to 643,000,963 pounds, being,
to make a round calculation, about thirty-three pounds yearly
for each individual then in the three kingdoms. The soap
used by manufacturers is not here included.

The description of society amongst whom plague still
exists, agrees exactly with what has been given. The disease
is very frequently observed to break out at Constantinople,
in that part of the city which is low and marshy, and there,
as every where else, nitidæ ædes haud æque facile infici-
untur ac sordidæ.—*City Remembrancer, Phil. Trans.* vol. vii.
At Aleppo, Dr. Russel says, " it always begins in the Keisa-
rias and Judidas : the former are small huts, with few or no
windows which stand crowded together, and are inhabited
by the lowest Arabs ; the latter, are the dwellings of the
inferior Jews, whose houses are small, or if large, the different apartments are crowded with different families. Many
of them are more than a story below the level of the street,
in a condition half ruinous, dirty in the extreme, damp, badly
aired, and the wretched inhabitants are clothed in rags."—
Concerning Grand Cairo, Savary asserts, " that its inhabitants are heaped together in thousands, and it is computed
that twenty inhabitants there, occupy a less space than one
inhabitant of London."—*Letters sur l'Egypt,* vol. iii. pp.
15-16. The description in the City Remembrancer, says,
" it is crowded by a vast number of inhabitants, who, for the
most part, live very meanly and nastily ; the streets are very
narrow and close, and twenty and thirty live together in one
small house. It is situated on a sandy plain at the foot of a
mountain, which, by keeping off the winds that would refresh
the air, makes the heats very stifling ; through the midst of
it passes a large canal, which is filled with water at the in-
flowing of the Nile, and after the river is decreased, is gradually dried up. Into this, people throw all manner of filth,
carrion, &c. so that the stench, which rises from this and the

mud together, is insufferably offensive. In this posture of
things, the plague every year constantly arises upon the inhabitants, and is only stopped when the Nile, by overflowing,
washes away this load of filth, the cold winds which set
in at the same time, lending their assistance by purifying the
air. We before said, on the authority of Assilini, that when
plague rages in Cairo, the citadel is free.

Algiers consists of a crowd of houses packed upon the
side of a steep hill, as if by accident. No stranger can look
at it from outside without wondering how he is to get in ;
and when he is within its gates the wonder is how he is to
get out. There is only one tolerable street, and even this is
not broad enough to allow two loaded camels to pass each
other without the foot-passengers stopping or standing aside.
If the load of a single camel happens to project a little from
its side, the biped is glad to stand squat against the wall,
and have the word " baylac" constantly resounding in his
ears. If he happen to walk slow, or be inattentive to the
warning voice, the big uncouth head of one of these brutes
will present itself over one of his shoulders before he knows
rightly where he is. The other streets are only about half
the breadth, and some of them very steep, and, as the houses
nearly meet at top, they have the appearance of dark, dirty
alleys. When viewed from the flat roofs of the houses, such
a street looks like a gutter between two dwellings, and the
hum of human voices below, and now and then a peep at a
stalking figure arrayed in white, are the only things which
undeceive the stranger.

Houses placed so closely to each other can never receive
much fresh air from the street, nor are the doors and windows
sufficiently numerous or large for this purpose, even if the
streets had been broader ; the dwellings, therefore, some of
which are large and even elegant within doors, receive light
and air from a court or square in the centre of the edifice.
Viewed from the top of a house, the whole town appears to
be a succession of these squares ; when the houses are high

they are more like deep pits; the eye cannot trace the lines of the streets, or observe openings of any other kind. Few of the streets have any thing like pavement; the drains are above ground, if any, and in the middle of the street. The houses, when viewed from the street, have the appearance of places built for defence; they are entered either by a large covered gateway, or a small narrow door, and a steep, narrow and very often a circular stair leads into the interior. A window or rather loop-hole is placed so as to give the inmates a view of the door, should any one apply for admittance; but there are few even of this kind of openings to the street. On one side of the door of each house, there is generally a depôt of ashes and dirt, which has been pushed out at an opening in the wall made for this purpose. The town is surrounded with a high wall, which has more the appearance of a church-yard wall than that of a fortified city. The ditch is always so dry, from the rocky bottom and sudden declivity, that the huts of the poorer class are built in it. The population at the time we visited it (which was a fortnight or three weeks before the arrival of the late French expedition) was reckoned at from 60 to 80,000. The venereal disease has long been treated here without mercury. Bread and raisins, we were told, constitutes the only diet of the patients. If we might judge from the mutilated faces, and the frequency of secondary symptoms, this regimen has not been very successful. Mr. Shultz, the Swedish Consul, who has been about thirty years at Algiers, informed us that plague appears every eight or ten years, and is generally believed to come in ships from Alexandria.

Tunis, Tripoli, Smyrna, and Alexandria, are so well known as to require no description. Alexis Tulin, Esq. the British Vice-Consul at Algiers, was at Tunis during the last great epidemic plague, and he and his family escaped an attack by shutting themselves up in their house. Mr. T. informed us that plague appeared in a family where the strictest quarantine had been enjoined. This could not be accounted for till

it was discovered that one of the iron bars of the window
was loose and had evidently been taken out for some purpose
or other. It was afterwards ascertained that this had been
done with a view to smuggle articles into the house.

It is a curious fact that, while a belief in contagion is
losing ground in this country, and when a question as to the
propriety and expediency of maintaining our present system
of quarantine against plague was brought into the British parliament, the Barbary and other Mahometan powers were opening their eyes to the dangers arising from free intercourse.
Both Mahomed Ally and Ibram Pacha, have become rational
contagionists; and Mr. Dickson, surgeon at Tripoli, told us
of his having succeeded in preventing the introduction of
plague by confining those ill of it on board their own vessels
in the harbour. This of course was done with the appro-
bation of the Bashaw.

The effects of crowding, filth, &c. are every way as well
exemplified by events in our maritime history. Improvements
have taken place at various times in the Royal Navy, with
regard to the healthy arrangements of our ships of war, and
the voyages of Lord Anson and Captain Cook contain lessons
which ought never to be forgotten. But it was chiefly under
the enlightened administrations of Earls St. Vincent and
Spencer, and the late Lord Melville, that the greatest improvements were adopted. The rigid discipline of a Jervis
proved every way as conspicuous in improving the health of
our ships, as the great fire of 1666 and the improvements
that succeeded it, did in banishing plague and other mortal
diseases from the first city of the empire.

The establishment of a sick berth, or hospital, to keep the
sick removed from the sound; the excellent arrangements of
ship's store-rooms to promote ventilation; cleanliness of men's
persons; cleaning of decks remote from ventilation by dry-
rubbing; correcting damp and foul air by burning fires; introducing seamen's dress suitable to the climate, and the airing
of beds and bedding when the weather would permit, were

all improvements which could not fail of having a powerful effect. Of such consequence was the latter practice considered by Earl St. Vincent, that he caused it to be inserted in ship's logs. There was no article in the public instructions issued to naval commanders respecting ventilation and cleanliness till the edition promulgated in 1806.

The general introduction of lime-juice into the Navy, forms a great era in its history. This was known as a remedy in scurvy nearly 200 years before, as appears from the following extract. " In the year 1600, Commodore Lancaster sailed from England on the 2nd of April with three other ships ; they arrived in Saldanha Bay on the 1st of August, the Commodore's crew being in perfect health, from the administration of three table-spoonfuls of lemon-juice every morning to each of his men ; whereas, the other ships were so sickly, that they were unmanageable for want of hands, and the commander was obliged to send men on board to take in their sails and hoist out their boats."—*Purchas's Pilgrim*, vol. i. p. 149. It is likewise mentioned in a work by Woodal, published in London in 1636, p. 165. The work is entitled the Surgeon's Mate.

But it was not till the year 1795, and during the distinguished administration of Earl Spencer, that an order for a general supply to the navy was accomplished in consequence of a representation from the Navy Medical Board. We have had no means of ascertaining what share the physicians at the head of the medical department of the navy had in these improvements ; but the names of Lind, Blane, Trotter, Gillespie, Harness, Weir, Burnett, Baird, Beatie, Dickson, Hutchison, Hammuk, Dobson, Johnson and Wilson, are sufficient to shew that the medical staff of the navy can boast of having had men as distinguished for talent, learning and assiduity, as that of any other department of the public service. Several men, who began their career in the navy, attained a high rank in their profession in after life—Kellie, Allan, and Lizars are amongst the number.

The late Lord Melville had the honour of being the first

statesman who raised the medical officers of the navy to a respectable rank in the service. Surgeons formerly found all their own medicines ; a gratuitous supply of the principal ones was directed in 1796, and an entire supply of them in 1804. These, with the increase of the seamen's pay, and other comforts, will long continue to distinguish the name of Melville in our naval annals, was there nothing else to make it be held in remembrance. Formerly each seaman and marine was allowed half a pint of rum daily ; this has been lately reduced to an imperial gill, and in lieu they are paid so much money every month. This is undoubtedly a great improvement ; as the men formerly had no money paid them on foreign stations, of course they had it not in their power to procure fruit and other little comforts. When they were granted leave to go on shore, the sailors sold their clothes to procure money. Much more care is now taken to keep the men from being disturbed during meals, or in their watches below.

The Hon. Sir Robert Spencer (whose death is deeply to be deplored) set a bright example in this. We have seen him holding the wheel, and his officers pulling at the ropes rather than disturb the men at their dinner hour. This is as it should be, for if there be no time in which a seaman can count on having a momentary independence, he is sure to become discontented and unhappy. The great importance of the improvements we have described soon became manifest. Sir Gilbert Blane affirms, that if the mortality during the twenty years revolutionary war had been equal to what it was in 1779, the whole stock of seamen would have been extinct ; and he computes, that two ships of war are capable of more service than three of the same rate in former times. " No longer do we hear," says Dr. Baird, " of ship-fever laying up ships of the line, and their services lost to the country for many months together."

Dr. Lind, in his book on the health of seamen, states that, from the 1st of July, 1758, to the 1st of July, 1760, no less than 2,174 were admitted into Haslar Hospital with fevers out of 5,743, for all that was taken in.—P. 141. It may give us some idea of the virulence of the contagion of fever in those days, to take another extract from his works. He says, "from a small spark of contagion once introduced into a fleet, and by the sick from that fleet into the town of Brest and its vicinity, more than 10,000 people, besides five physicians, 150 surgeons, and 200 almoners and nurses, fell victims to its rage, with many slaves, who, by a promise of their liberty, were engaged to assist the sick."

It appears from the Appendix to Dr. Sinclair's Thesis, published in Edinburgh in 1817, that, during the years 1810,11 and 12, there were sent to the naval hospital at Malta, Gibraltar, and Minorca, from our fleets employed in the Mediterranean and Adriatic, the crews of which were computed at 15,000 men, 590 cases of pulmonary affection, 1,242 cases of fever, and 169 of dysentery. The excellent practical work of Sir William Burnett, ascribes a great proportion of the fevers that prevail in our fleets in this quarter of the world to marsh miasmata. The number of cases of dysentery was here very small. From the abstract of the official returns of the whole army employed in the Peninsula, from December, 1811, to June, 1814, it appears that nearly 23,000 cases of dysentery and diarrhoea occurred in that period of thirty-one months.—Vide *Luscombe on the Health of Soldiers*, pp. 4 and 38.

According to the following tables, the average rate of the mortality of the British navy, for the three last years of the late war, was one in 30·25. There were on board ships in all parts of the world—

	Number.	Died.
On the 1st January, 1811	108,581	5,183
—————————— 1812	136,778	4,265
—————————— 1813	138,324	4,211

But these tables include those who were killed, drowned, &c. ; and Sir Gilbert Blane thinks there are good reasons for believing that violent deaths constitute about one half of the mortality on board ships of war.—Vide *Blane's Dissertations*.

The average mortality of the navy, therefore, in this report, from sickness, is only 1 in 61; whereas, the average mortality for the whole of England, as taken from the parliamentary returns of 1811, was 1 in 48·7; London, 1 in 38; and in the year 1811, Liverpool was 1 in 30, so that the navy at the same period, was in reality twice as healthy as the latter place. The majority of sailors, it is true, are men in the prime of life; but it is just such men that are most liable to fevers, particularly in hot climates, where a great proportion of them were then serving:—and when the privations they are obliged to undergo, and the hardships and dangers to which they are constantly exposed, are taken into the account; when it is considered that 590 men are cooped up in a seventy-four gun ship; that most of these men sleep upon one deck, each having only fourteen inches for his hammock; that for a great part of their time they have nothing but salted provisions; sometimes only half allowance of food in a putrid state, with a small proportion of water, which is likewise stinking; that they frequently change from cold climates to hot ones, and from hot to cold ones in a few weeks; and that at all times they are liable to be harrassed by night as well as by day, and exposed to every kind of weather, often without the possibility of providing against it; we say, when all these things are duly considered, the conclusion is irresistible, that the British Navy is as deservedly famous for its internal polity, as it undoubtedly is in war.

The health of the French army in Egypt, offers another remarkable proof of what can be done by a great and enlightened people in preventing disease. The report of the minister of war (Berthier), to the Consuls of the French Republic, dated 4th April, 1801, contains the following statement:—"In Europe, during the war, the number of sick was to that of effective men as 1 to 12; and before the revolution, during peace, the proportion was the same. In Egypt, it has been during the month of brumaire (October, November), as 1 to 28; and during frimaire (Novem-

ber, December), as 1 to 30. In Europe, in the military hospitals, the number of deaths is to that of sick admitted
during the month, as 1 to 23 ; in Egypt, during the month
of brumaire, the proportion has commonly been as 1 to 43 ;
and in frimaire, as 1 to 37. The increase of deaths during
this last month, was owing to the contagious disease ; which,
though little spread, was beginning to show itself.

" It is known, that in Europe, the number of sick is to the
population, as 1 to 20 ; and that in a month, the mortality is
to the number of sick, as 1 to 19 ; so that the best established facts prove, that *the climate of Egypt* is already
become to Frenchmen more healthy than their *native country,*
or than any other country in Europe. What then will it be
when the sciences and arts shall have diffused all their advantages, and shall have banished from it its contagious
diseases, and instructed us in the means of preventing the
ophthalmy."—Vide *Assilini, p.* 203. When we compare the
state of such an army with that of Ibram Pacha, which our
sailors in the Morea jocularly baptised "the one-eyed corps,"
we cannot be surprised at the superior health and efficiency
of the former.

But amongst the many instances recorded of the happy
effects of proper government on the health of mankind, that
of the late Duke of Kent, in Gibraltar, stands pre-eminent.
" This garrison," according to Sir James Fellowes, " had for
a length of time been visited by a considerable number of
deaths every year ; but in the time his Royal Highness had
the command, the deaths were reduced to one-fourth *of the
usual mortality of private life." ! !—Reports.*

There is still one branch of the public service that deserves being mentioned here, viz. the management of our
convict ships—where virtue and principle are wanting, the
task must be more arduous.

In Collins' History of New South Wales, pp. 102 and 436,
it is stated, that a contract had been entered into by Government, with Messrs. Calvert, Cambden, and King, merchants

in London, for the transporting 1,000 convicts, and Government engaged to pay 17*l.* 7*s.* 6*d.* per head for every convict embarked. This sum being as well for their provisions as for their transportation, no interest for their preservation was created in the owners, &c. The following account of the numbers who died on board each ship, was given by the masters :—On board of Julian, five women and two children died ; in the Surprise, forty-two men ; Scarborough, sixty-eight men ; and on board the Neptune, one hundred and fifty-one men, eleven women, and two children ; so that two hundred and sixty-one men, sixteen women, and four children died, making the whole mortality two hundred and eighty-one. If all the men and women were included in the number of one thousand convicts, the mortality in about *four months*, the time of the passage, was little less than 1 in $3\frac{1}{2}$; a sentence of transportation during such a state of things, was worse in some respects than one for immediate execution. On board the Hillsborough, which arrived on the 26th July, 1799, ninety-five died during the passage, and six men after they were landed.—*Ibid.* " Within the period since naval surgeons have been appointed to convict ships, and better regulations with regard to ventilation, cleanliness, and crowding adopted, it is considered very unfortunate indeed if *two or three* deaths occur in a voyage. Out of 1,059 convicts that were embarked in England and Ireland, 1,057 were landed at Sydney, in tolerable good health."—Vide *Two Voyages to New South Wales, &c. by Thomas Reid, surgeon, R. N. (London,* 1822), *pp.* 281-2. The average mortality where crowding and filth existed, was 1 in $3\frac{1}{2}$; but where better regulations were adopted, it was 1 in 500.

Sydenham, who fled from the plague of 1663, and who remarked, that fevers constituted two-thirds of mortal diseases, and that eight out of nine of all who died, were cut off by them, was misled by a wrong theory. Had he formed more correct notions of their causes and been equally successful in their prevention, the sum of human misery must

N

have been prodigiously lessened. But, if Sydenham and the physicians of that age were somewhat in fault for not taking due advantage of the knowledge of their time, what must be the errors of those philosophers of the present day who would willingly sell the dear-bought experience of so many ages for a mouthful of words. That contagion has been generated under such circumstances as we have described cannot well be doubted. Let us examine a few of the facts and arguments that have been put forth in support of a contrary doctrine.

It has been said that none of the cases of crowding, filth, &c. related by authors, afford any thing like a *direct* proof that contagion was ever generated by such means. This is so far correct. All that we know is, that contagious diseases have, in all ages, been observed to arise and prevail under such circumstances of crowding and filth. On the other hand, they rarely exist where ventilation and cleanliness are strictly enforced. Remove the evident causes of contagious diseases and the diseases themselves will become extinct.

The next mode by which the doctrine has been assailed is negative proof, a kind of evidence which has been deservedly considered as inadmissible in all judicial proceedings, when any of the ordinary affairs of life became the subjects of investigation. Because A did not attack B at such a time and place, is no evidence that A did not assault C at another time and place. Neither would a thousand instances of honesty in John be received as proof that John, who had stolen a sheep, was not a thief, nor would *direct* proof be required to convict him, for there might be presumptive evidence of his guilt that no judge or jury could refuse. For example, if sheep were frequently stolen when John was present, and never when he was absent, we believe there are few rational persons who would not try to save their flocks, by banishing John as soon as possible. But this is not the only objection we have to the negative evidence adduced on the present question.

Dr. Bancroft, who may be regarded as the Agamemnon of his sect, and who has shown much tact in selecting bits of evidence which suited his theory, while he leaves behind the pieces which are less palatable, has also dealt largely in negative evidence, and he has brought forward several instances where crowding, filth, &c. have failed in generating contagion. We have already had occasion to find fault with this species of plum-picking, much more with the arguments founded upon it. At pages 105-6, he says, "No accidental collection, nor even the most artificial and scientific combination of either organic or inorganic matters, not impregnated with specific contagion, could create contagion." In the above passage the Doctor is quite correct, for the idea of accidental or even artificial means being adequate to form a contagion in the way we cook a custard, or make a cataplasm, is too absurd to deserve a moment's consideration. We could no more expect putrid animal and vegetable substances to generate a contagion or morbid secretion out of the body, than we could suppose such substances in the shape of human food to form blood without passing through the digestive process in the animal system. Amongst his negative proof he brings forward asphyxia, or "almost immediate death," from being suddenly exposed to the vapours arising from privies, &c. p. 113. "But such mischiefs," he adds, "have no relation to fever." What then is the value of this proof? The fever is the creative power which generates contagion during disease, in the same way the digestive process is required to convert food into blood during health; that the products of putrefaction, when not sufficiently concentrated and powerful to occasion "almost immediate death," sometimes, particularly when long applied in ill-ventilated and confined places, cause fever, and that that fever has in many instances proved to be contagious, we have before shown.

Our ignorance of the modus operandi of such matters on such occasions, has likewise been brought forward as an objection by Dr. B. (pp. 120-1) but this is no stronger presumption against the generation of contagion by such means, than the fact of our not being able to explain in what manner the vital powers operate in converting our food into chyle and the chyle into blood.

Another part of the author's negative proof is made up of dead bodies putrefying *in the open air*; and at p. 117, he says, " if the exhalations from piles of bodies destroyed by the plague itself and corrupting *in the open air* were thus incapable of generating the contagion, either of fever or of plague, even during the prevalence of a pestilential consti-tution of the atmosphere (if any state of the atmosphere ever deserved that title), it may, I think, be safely affirmed, that there are no circumstances under which putrid animal matter can be supposed ever to produce febrile contagion." This is another case that cannot warrant the important conclusion drawn from it. The *dead* bodies while undergoing rapid decomposition in the open air could not be expected to per-form the functions of *living ones*, or throw out from their surfaces the pestilential contagion, as they had done before death. If they failed to emit the contagion by which life had been destroyed, it was surely less likely that they would generate febrile contagion. The effects of the exhalations arising from them on those who were exposed to their in-fluence would depend on the time they were exposed, the circumstances under which they were exposed, the state of their health at the time, and many other circumstances of which we have no means of judging. Dr. Bancroft's nega-tive proof, founded on the crowding and filth of persons in health, is not more conclusive.

We have already shewn the dependance of all the con-tagions on temperature and other circumstances connected with climate and season; and we have likewise pointed out how far Dr. B. is a believer in such influence. One particular dogma of his, it will be recollected, is, that typhus contagion cannot operate, nor even exist, in a tropical climate; another is, that the contagion of plague is destroyed, either by great heat or by great cold. Now, if these contagions *when formed* be so very dependant on temperature, it is surely not unreasonable to conclude that both the extremes of heat and cold must likewise prevent their generation. These reflections, however, do not hinder the Doctor from travelling so far out of his way as the Frigid Zone on one side, and the burning shores of Africa on the other, in order to collect his negative proof. Accordingly the Russians, Greenlanders, Kamstchatkans and Esquimaux, are the first people that strike his fancy. We are not sufficiently well acquainted with the manners and customs of those people to speak positively concerning them, and if we were, our limits would prevent us from enlarging on the subject. We should, however, imagine that a four-posted bedstead of ice, with pillows and curtains of the same *raw* material, would not be so liable to imbibe and collect the effluvia arising from the bodies of the Esquimaux, even if the same quantity of effluvium was emitted from their surface in so cold a climate; nor would the effluvium and other kinds of filth be so liable to decomposition and recomposition. 2nd. The houses (if they can be called so) of the other people, lined with moss, and perpetually obscured in columns of smoke arising from fires made of the same antiseptic material, might be supposed, without any great stretch of imagination, to have some effect in counteracting the bad effects arising from human effluvia. 3rd. The temperate lives of the people themselves, render them less liable to acute diseases, although, in the season of their confinement within doors, they are universally affected with scurvy. Query; does not this scorbutic taint counteract, or even destroy the susceptibility to fever? 4th. The Russians make large use of an antiseptic chink called *quass*, to which Dr. Matthew Guthrie, physician at St. Petersburg, attributes their non-liability to putrid fever. —Vide *Letter to Dr. Priestly, in the* 68*th* vol. *Phil. Trans.* Lastly, the practice of bathing, so common in Russia, deserves to be taken into the account. Upon the whole, we cannot see how any thing like a fair inference can be drawn from Dr. B.'s evidence in the Polar regions.

Negative proof derived from the crowding of Negroes on board of slave-ships is liable to many objections. If it be true that neither typhus nor plague could exist in the great heat of the African coast, and that yellow fever is not contagious, but a disease arising from marsh miasmata, and one to which Negroes are not liable, as Dr. B. affirms, is it fair to adduce negative evidence from such a source? The very fact of the author condescending on such evidence, appears to us a strong presumption, nay, an almost direct acknowledgment of his incapacity to find less objectionable proof. There are, besides, many circumstances in the condition of Negroes on board of slave-ships, which render them less liable to be affected by human effluvium. Without clothes to collect and retain it on the surface, it is no sooner emitted than it is dissipated by the sun and winds. Their skins, as before noticed, are well adapted to the keeping up of a free perspiration, of course to prevent the occurrence of febrile heat, while their regular, temperate lives, render them less susceptible of acute and inflammatory diseases. The situation of convicts during a voyage to New South Wales is very different. The convict sails from a country where typhus contagion may be generated, but passes on a voyage of much greater length through climates where it may still exist; he is confined to the society of a people amongst whom it oftenest originates, and he has been banished from his native land, partly on account of those irregular and dissolute habits which predispose him to disease. Let us here give a short account of a case of this kind. The breaking out of the yellow fever on board the ship Hankey, at Bulama, in 1792, forms a great era in the history of that disease. It has likewise been rendered famous by the accounts given of it by different authors, but particularly by Dr. Chisholm, on the side of contagion, and by Dr. Bancroft on the opposite, in his seventh Appendix; which has been looked upon by some of the miasmatics as every way as destructive to the doctrine of contagion in yellow fever as Buonaparte's Berlin and Milan decrees were formerly expected to be to British commerce. The ship Hankey sailed from Gravesend on the 4th of April, 1792, in company with the Calypso and Beggar's Bennison. In the Calypso, a vessel of 298 tons, 149 colonists for Bulama, including thirty-six women and thirty-one children, were embarked, in all, with officers, 155 persons; on board the Hankey of 260 tons, 123, of whom twenty-six were women and twenty-six children; in the sloop of thirty-four tons, six persons: making in all 284, including seventy-two women and fifty-seven children, besides the crews of the vessels, the peoples' large quantity of baggage, provisions, ships' stores, and furnishings for a new settlement in a distant and uninhabited island.

Captain Beaver, in different parts of his African Memoranda, and in a letter published in Wadstrom's Essay, p. 300, speaks of these people as little better than the sweepings of the jails of the metropolis, and of course the very dregs of society. In the letter, he says, " they were habituated to drunkenness, idleness, and all the vices of the capital, most of whom came here (to Bulama) in dread of punishment from crimes committed against their country's laws;" and he calls the Hankey " the noisy, dirty, disorderly Hankey;" so that the whole scheme cannot be looked upon in any other light than a genteel mode of transportation, and the people as convicts, but with this important difference, that they were banished to a country not previously comfortably settled, but one in which they were doomed to undergo a train of misfortunes, perhaps unexampled in the history of colonization.

These unfortunate people, unaccustomed to sea and to the confined and crowded decks of a ship, experienced many privations during a tedious stormy passage to a hot climate, without proper medical aid in case of sickness, without the means of keeping themselves clean, and without the taste or inclination to do so, even if they had possessed such means.

The yellow fever appeared on board the Hankey when she was at anchor in sight of the place of destination, and before the colonists on board of her had landed. Such is a short description of this celebrated case. We shall again revert to it, and treat it more fully in our review of the evidence on the nature of yellow fever. In the meantime, we shall only remark that, he who would question the possibility of contagion arising under such circumstances, must be but little acquainted with its history; it is at least a very different case, in many important particulars, from the crowding of Negroes on board of slave-ships.

Dr. Bancroft allows that yellow fever has broken out in ships at sea when placed under similar circumstances; but here, as in the case of the fever at Bulama, he flies to marsh-miasmata, which he thinks is generated by the foul ballast, stinking bilgewater, and the filthiness of these vessels generally. The following passage extracted from a book on West India fever, written by Dr. Wilson, surgeon of the Royal Navy, would, however, lead us to believe, that Dr. B. has lately so far abandoned his favourite theory. Doctor Wilson's words are these :—" Dr. Bancroft, whose labours in this field are so well-known and so highly appreciated, who has collected so much information and exhibited so much talent to prove that this disease (yellow fever) depends on earthy exhalations for its cause as entirely as does intermittent fever, finds *the whole of his elaborate and highly-finished structure sapped* by the fever in the Iphigenia; he finds here a stumbling-block which he had not expected and cannot *remove, and he freely confesses the insuperable nature of the difficulty.*"

Before leaving this subject, it is necessary to point out some material differences that exist between marsh and morbid poisons. The first is formed from dead organised matter out of the body; the second is a morbid secretion, and therefore can only be produced by an act of the animal system. The same degrees of heat, moisture, air and rest, will uniformly act the same way on dead organised matter of the same kind and under the same circumstances; and for this reason, that such matter has no power within itself of resisting external agents, and, as these agents are uniformly regulated by the same laws, the result of their operation must be uniformly the same. This is not the case with living organised matter, and for this reason, that living animals and plants, possess a power within themselves of resisting, altering, or modifying the influence of external stimuli. For example, the same stage of fermentation in certain vegetable substances, will always produce vinegar, saccharine matter, or wine, according as circumstances are altered: but the same quantity of alcohol will not always have the same effect on the human body, neither will water at a certain temperature; for water at forty-five degrees of Fahrenheit, will produce a sensation of heat at one time, and a sensation of cold in a short time afterwards on *the same person*. Again, dead matter, when placed in an oven heated to the 160th degree, will soon acquire a like temperature, but the animal body under such circumstances will retain its natural heat—thus, a living dog can resist a heat that would roast him if dead. If the animal body, then, has a power so to alter and modify the effects of external agents, and if this power be so very different at one time from what it is at other times, what can be the value of a few cases where crowding and filth proved insufficient to generate febrile contagion ? Many instances have occurred of persons falling down in a fit of apoplexy and dying suddenly, merely from immersing their feet in cold water. Ten thousand instances of this practice proving harmless, could never do away with the simple fact that such immersion was the cause of death. In the last case, it is true, we can understand how death is produced, consequently no one disputes the fact; but we cannot explain in what manner crowding and filth, under certain circumstances, cause fevers, which afterwards spread by contagion, consequently, there is room left for speculation and doubt.

Nature of Contagion—Mode of Spreading, &c.

The nature of contagion has not yet been accurately ascertained; although, so far as its prevention is concerned, our knowledge of it cannot be considered as unimportant. In the age when microscopic observations were more fashionable than they are at present, many, if not all of the contagions were ascribed to vermination by physiologists and pathologists. Even Shakespeare alludes to this, and says, " What ! sigh for the tooth-ache, which is but an humour or a *worm.*" The school of Linnæus was, however, the most remarkable for this doctrine, though it has not been confined to that seminary. Linnæus himself, laboured hard to prove that dysentery is the effect of a peculiar larve or grub belonging to the acarus or tick genus, which he has ventured to introduce into his Natural History under the name of *Acarus Dysenteriæ.* In like manner, Kitcher has ascribed the plague to another kind of animalcule ; Langius, the measles ; various others the itch ; Sigier, petechiæ ; Lusitanus and Poncellus, small-pox ; De Suult, canine madness ; Hauptman, syphilis ; Martin and Udonan, both pupils of Linnæus, elephantiasis ; and Nyander, another pupil of the same great master, contagious diseases of most, if not of all kinds. Others have ascribed to the same cause, piles, tooth-ache, and even the inspissated and vermiform mucus squeezed out occasionally from the excretory ducts of the small mucous glands of the forehead, in the present system described under the genus and species *Ionthus Varus.* Vide *for Exanthemata Viva in Amenitat. Academ.* vol. v. p. 90— also, *Study of Medicine,* vol. i. p. 291. As to the opinions of the older authors regarding the origin of epidemics, it may be said, tot capita, tot sensus. It may be observed, however, that a belief in aerial causes was the most general. Thus Hippocrates, de natura hominis et de flatibus, ascribes the origin of malignant fevers to terrestrial exhalations and vitiation of the air. Galen, lib. 1, De Dies. Febr. c. vi. says, "In pestilenti æris statu, inspiratio potissimum febris causa est :" and Sydenham, admits the same thing in his book, Obs. de Morbis Acutis, 1, cap. 1.

Dionysius, of Halicarnassus, Antiq. Rom. lib. vii., relates, that the Volsci suffered a dreadful epidemic, caused by the exhalations of the Pontine Marshes ; but that this historian was aware of contagion in some epidemics, we have before shown.

Paulo Alexandri and Nicolas Massa, attributed the plague of Venice in 1535, to the fetid exhalations of the canals which form the streets of that city. Philippe Ingrassia, Informazione del Pestifero Morbo de Palermo, says, that the continual rains of 1557, occasioned so terrible a disease in the capital of Sicily, that, in five months, nearly 8,000 people died there.

Baccio Baldini, in his commentary on the book of Hippocrates, De Ære Aquis et Locis, blames the inundations of a river to the east of Florence. Andrea Gratiola, Discorso di Peste, does not hesitate to assert, that the corrupt waters of the canals of Venice frequently produced there, petechial fevers, and other fevers of a bad character.

Placentino, De Peste, cap. vi., relates, that a cruel epidemic devastated the town of Nola, in Calabria, which he attributes to the putrid exhalations arising from the plain on which it is built. Sylvius de le Boe thought that the plague of Leyden was caused by the stagnant waters of the canals which traverse and environ that city. Forestus gave the same reason for the epidemics of Delft and Leyden. Lancisi, De Nox. Palud. Effluv., relates, that the epidemic which raged at Rome, in 1696, was caused by the stagnant waters of the ditches of the Castle Saint Ange, and of the meadows at the foot of Monte Mazio. Ramazzini attributes the epidemic which ravaged the plain of Modena, in 1680, to the putrid exhalations of the waters which sojourn there ; and Gollich, Ephraim, Olde, &c. gave the same origin to the epidemics of

Cleves, in 1720, and of Cullembourg, in 1761. The opinions above stated, will serve to show that an endemic origin was frequently given to contagious diseases, as well as marsh fevers. We shall add a few other notions that have been entertained by different authors.

Volcanos (Portius); earthquakes (Messaria, &c. &c.); comets and the openings of caverns, from which poisonous vapours exhale (Zacchias); mineral exhalations (Arburthnot); cold (Riverius); excessive heat (Pringle and Hoffman); dryness (Diemerbroeck); the rains (Degorter); sudden changes of the seasons (Sauvages); calmness (Gostaldi); the dews (Pajati); the fogs or mists (Portius); the south wind (Sauvages).

In fine, says Ozanam, Histoire Medicale des Maladies Epidemiques, Contagieuses et Epizootiques, vol. i. p. 21, they have accused the elements, metals, minerals, and the creatures themselves, phlagiston, oxygen, carbonic acid, azot, and hydrogen, predominating in the atmosphere.

The terms endemic, epidemic, contagious and infectious, it will be seen, have been differently used by authors, and strangely confounded by many. " By the first," Dr. Adams says, "we understand diseases which are known only in certain places, often only in certain latitudes, where they are found *in every season;*" by epidemic, he " understands those which occur only in certain seasons, or other changes in the atmosphere, of the nature of which we are unacquainted, or from contagion : the first order for the most part are chronic, the second, acute diseases." According to this definition, if we understand it rightly, marsh poison is not an endemic cause, for it frequently does not exist in places *in every season*, nor are the diseases it excites always properly termed *chronic diseases.* As marsh fevers sometimes occur in certain places only at certain seasons, and produce acute diseases, they fall under the class of epidemics, at least as he defines the terms. Under endemics, Dr. A. classes leprosy, elephantiasis, and some diseases which he owns are considered by some as contagious. But whether they be contagious or not, they cannot, strictly speaking, fall under the class of endemics, even according to his own definition ; for, although they are known to prevail more in some places than in others, they have no necessary connexion with locality, any more than scurvy has with a particular ship. According to our view, therefore, they are *statistical diseases*, depending more on the manners and customs of the people than on any thing connected with the locality. The author's mode of classifying contagious diseases with those arising from general atmospheric causes, seems calculated to lead to very erroneous and confused notions concerning them. It serves, in fact, to perpetuate the very errors that most, if not all, of the authors whose names we have mentioned above have committed ; for few or none of them seem to have considered the contagions as strictly statistical or artificial causes. We have before noticed the distinction made between contagion and infection in the senses in which they are used by Dr. Adams.

In order to avoid, if possible, some of these errrors, we have divided all the causes of disease into two grand classes, viz. *natural*, and *artificial* or *statistical*. The first class comprehends those *causes arising from natural objects, or inseparably connected with the performance of natural functions.* It, therefore, includes two orders of causes :—1st. *Those natural to the human body as depending on the performance of necessary functions.* Under this order, birth, growth, dentition, age, sex, temperament and idiosyncrasy, and decay, as also the sexual causes, menstruation, parturition, labour, and periodical changes, fall to be considered. The second order of natural causes, we have called *topographical*, for the want of a better term, and the definition is—*causes arising from natural objects unconnected with the body ;* this order we subdivide into *general* and *local.* Under the *general causes,* air, water, caloric, light, the electric fluid, meteors, and their connexion with climate, season, and weather, as winds, rains, dews, fogs, &c. fall to be noticed. The *local causes* comprehend in their consideration, situation, soil, cultivation, natural productions, mountains, woods, lakes, rivers, marshes, minerals, &c. &c.

The *statistical causes* are " *those arising from human actions.*" Of these we have made five orders, and we put the contagions under the third, viz.—" *causes arising from congregation and intercourse.*" Of this order there are five genera, *viz.* contagion, hereditary taint or disposition, sympathy, imitation and habit. The contagions are divided into *those communicated by touch ;* as itch, syphilis, gonorrhœa, sibbins, yaws, elephantiasis, plica, scald-head, herpes, ringworm, ophthalmia, cow-pox, hydrophobia, &c. 2nd. *Those communicated by contact or near approach ;* small-pox, chicken-pox, scarlet fever, measles, cholera, and hooping-cough. 3rd. *Those acute contagions which are more dependant on climate ;* plague, typhus, yellow and puerperal fever.* Such is our view of the causes of diseases connected with the present subject : the others have been noticed under their proper heads. It would not be a difficult task to point out some defects in this arrangement also ; we do not offer it as perfect. For example, temperament and idiosyncrasy, being often transmitted lineally, they perhaps more properly belong to the second genus of the order of causes which arise from congregation and intercourse, *viz.* hereditary taint or influence. Woods and mountains are only causes of diseases, in so far as they obstruct the free circulation of air and water ; and cultivation of the soil may be said to come under the head of statistical causes, as depending on human actions. Still we think the arrangement has one merit which no other we have seen possesses—that of pointing out to the general reader how much health depends upon human conduct, and how easily many of the most for-

* The division of the contagions is nearly the same as that made by Professor Hosack.

midable of our maladies may be prevented by proper care and management.

Several philosophers, both in France and England, have bestowed much pains in their researches into the nature of contagion, but unfortunately without success; the opinions entertained are, therefore, little to be depended upon. Some think it consists of a putrid ferment, others of azot and hydrogen, while a third set maintain its alkaline nature. It was from an idea of its alkaline nature, we believe, that acids were first used in the cure of contagious distempers, with a view of neutralizing the poison. It has besides been discovered, that the fumes of different acids destroyed the properties of contagious effluvia, and it has been believed by some, that they do so by imparting to them a portion of oxygen gas; this opinion is rendered more probable by finding that these acids act in this respect with an influence corresponding in degree to the facility with which they part with oxygen. From this it would appear that their anti-pestilential powers are in consequence of an union effected between the contagious matter and the oxygen gas they contain, by which the properties of the former are entirely altered. It has been presumed from these circumstances that oxygen entered sparingly into the composition of contagious vapour; an opinion which likewise appears to be confirmed by our knowledge that this matter is entirely or in greater part evolved from animal matters, into whose composition oxygen enters but in a small proportion. The composition of contagion, according to Fourcroy, consists of sulphuretted and phosporetted hydrogen gases, either in whole or in greater part; but it is thought by some that most of the elementary matters of the body also enter into its composition, and that a peculiar matter is thus generated, varying in its nature according to the number and proportion of matters composing it.

In the works of Dr. Wintringham, mention is made of the matter of a pestilential bubo having been examined by distillation, but without any satisfactory result. This cannot surprise us, when we consider how little is known of the nature of the blood and other animal fluids.

When contagion is held by other substances than the human body, those containing it are termed *fomites*. Were it not through the medium of other substances, epidemical diseases must have been much rarer in their appearance and more limited in their range, and it is chiefly by them that all the morbid poisons are collected, fostered and preserved from the destroying power of other agents. Dr. Cullen thought that contagion, propagated by means of fomites, was more virulent than by approximation to a contagious person. Such substances, when strongly impregnated with concentrated contagious effluvia, which have just emanated from the bodies of the sick, may in fact be compared to glasses which in-crease the heat by concentrating and collecting the calorific rays of the sun into a focus. Had the contagions not been provided with such places of refuge to protect them from other agents, their existence must have been more precarious; but, even with such aids, we are convinced that they must long ere this have become extinct, had they never been re-produced by matters dissimilar to themselves.

According to Fracastorius, " the matters best fitted to convey contagion, are such as are least liable to undergo any alteration in their composition, in consequence of the affinity of the contagion to the body itself, or from the effects of heat or moisture, or the powers of the whole united." The correctness of this observation must be evident to every one; for substances which are so very liable to undergo chemical changes themselves, can never be well fitted to preserve others from decomposition. Another thing must be just as evident, namely, that the fitness of a substance for acting as a fomites, depends greatly on its porosity. If the interstitial distances of its particles, are either too large or too minute, it cannot be so well adapted as matters whose interstitial foramina are of a medium size; in the one case, the admission of contagious effluvia is altogether prevented, and in the other, it is more apt to be excluded by the atmosphere or vapours of a different kind. Woollen clothes, agreeable to these principles, ought to be of all other substances the best calculated for retaining, collecting, and preserving contagion. Furs, feathers, old cotton goods, new cotton cloth, old linen, new linen, old silk, new silk, are probably so in their order; hemp, flax, tow, hair, shamois leather, paper, decayed timber, old lime walls, dry powders that are not susceptible of chemical change, and such like matters, are better fitted than stone, coal, metal, polished marble, glass, or bark, green wood, ripe fruits, or recent vegetables. On the same principle, the naked surface of a man exposed to the air is not so likely to accumulate and retain human or contagious effluvia as the clothed European, and a dead body undergoing rapid decomposition in the open air, can never prove infectious in the same way it had done before death. In this last case, the body has not only lost the power of secreting contagion, as it has done that of performing every living function, but the contagious effluvia that might be supposed to adhere to its surface at death, have to encounter the powerful operation of the sun, wind, and rain, on the one hand, and the chemical agents let loose by putrefaction on the other.

There may, however, be some cases where the products of putrefaction prove harmless in this way. It may give us some idea of the facility with which substances become impregnated with animal matters, to instance the case of the blood-hound in the chace. The hare and stag run with surprising quickness over a large space of ground, and although a foot touches any one part of that ground for an almost inconceivable short space of time, and the other parts of the bodies of these animals are at some distance from it, yet they leave behind them certain animal matters which enable the blood-hound to follow in their tract with wonderful exactness. Should the tracts of other animals cross their path, or even run nearly in a parallel direction with it, the

o

blood-hound is able to distinguish the difference between the scent or smell of the one from that of the other. We believe a dog can follow Its master in this way for many miles, though a considerable time may have elapsed since he travelled the road.

If substances be so readily impregnated with animal matter in the *open air*, from so small a surface as the body of a hare, in so short a time, and yet retain the smell imparted to them so long, how much more will blankets be impregnated, in which a sick person (or even a healthy one) has lain for months in a filthy, close, confined apartment, where fresh air is seldom, if ever permitted to enter. Yet, compare even this last case with the description of the houses of the poor in London, before quoted from the work of Dr. Willan, where six or seven individuals live in one apartment and sleep in one bed.

When clothes or blankets are kept in close places, as in a chest or trunk, they will of course retain contagious effluvia a much longer time. Such a chest may be compared to the air-tight phial which preserves even the most subtle and volatile drug from being destroyed by the action of other agents. Forestus gives an account of a pestilence having been again excited, by a person accidentally shaking and moving about some clothes that had been laid up some time in a chest, and which had been impregnated with the semina of that disease. Zonini mentions the case of a man, who was suddenly killed by a vapour which issued from a trunk, on opening it on board of a Turkish man-of-war, having the plague on board as it lay in the old harbour of Alexandria, in 1780. This last case may have been asphyxia only, yet it serves the purpose for which we quote it, namely, to show how well adapted close places are for retaining noxious effluvia. The fact, too, will explain how plague and yellow fever have sometimes been conveyed from place to place by ships, the crews of which were healthy. In the case of the Hankey at Grenada, in 1793, the clothes, beds and bedding, of the people who had died of yellow fever at the Island of Bulama and elsewhere, were discovered concealed in chests in the hold of that ill-fated vessel.

In the year 1511, Fracastorius relates that, when the Germans had possession of Verona, a great plague arose, which proved fatal to 10,000 men. He adds, " Ex una veste pellicea, non pauciores quam quinque et viginti Teutones obiise, uno defuncto alius enduebat vestem, et hoc alius, et alius donec monefacti tot defunctis vestem combuscere." This leathern vest or garment, which killed no fewer than twenty-five persons who wore it successively, must have become more impregnated with pestilential effluvia from each succeeding wearer. Had this fomes at last been closely locked up in a chest, the contagion might have been preserved for a length of time. A remarkable instance of the bad effects arising from fomites, is mentioned by Lind, Chap. IV. Sec. 11. In the year 1776, when the French squadron, under the command of the Duc d'Anville, passed the Summer at Chebucto, now Halifax, an infectious fever prevailed amongst them, and cut off a great number of their men. On the return of the squadron to Europe, several blankets and old clothes, which had been used in their tents and hospitals, were unfortunately left behind. These fatal receptacles of disease were soon after eagerly picked up by a party of Mimack Indians, who, in their wandering, chanced to visit the spot; they naturally clothed themselves with some of them, while they carried home others and distributed among their tribe; the unhappy consequence of which, were the almost total extinction of the Mimack nation, few of them having survived.

When the English traversed the country from Annapolis Royal, next Summer, they were surprised at seeing the dead bodies and skeletons of whole families lying unburied in their huts, until they were informed by the neutrals, who also inhabit that country, and the neighbouring Indians, that the Mimacks had been cut off by the French blankets; the

o 2

blankets were found in several of their huts, where not one
of the family remained.

Dr. Willan observes, that though the scarlet fever, when
epidemic in London, may have sometimes been imported
from abroad by means of infected goods, yet it will, he
thinks, be most frequently found to have originated in the
large repositories of old clothes, near the Tower and Smith-
field and Ratcliffe Highway. Therefore, the disease has
often begun in the *eastern* extremity of London and spread
westward. " During my last year's attendance at the Public
Dispensary," says he—" I had reason to think that a family
residing in Wild-street, Lincoln's Inn-fields, was affected
with scarlatina maligna, by clothes bought in Monmouth-
street. More than fifty persons in the adjoining houses were
soon infected with the disease, which afterwards traversed
Drury Lane, and spread by Long Acre and the streets connected with it—through several parishes in Westminster."—
On Cut. Dis. p. 391.

A contagious disease spreading more in one direction than
in others, has often been mentioned by authors as proof of
atmospheric influence. Dr. O'Halleran, one of the latest
authors on yellow fever, lays great stress on the epidemic of
Barcelona, in 1821, spreading from the eastern towards the
western parts of that city, but stopping after it had pro-
ceeded a certain length in this direction. The Doctor (like
many of the non-contagionists who have the winds at their
command on all occasions) thinks this fact quite conclusive
against contagion in that disease. Now it so happened, that
the good people of Barcelona had determined in former times
on making the streets of that city extremely narrow, and the
houses crowded, filthy and ill-ventilated; but, in course of
time, they discovered the inconvenience of such a mode of
building, and at last thought of forming wider streets and
larger and better-aired houses. It also happened, that the
older part of the city is further east than the other parts, so
that in every succeeding age, the streets built in the west got

broader and broader, the houses keeping pace with the streets in size and elegance. It moreover happened, that the rich dons and proud aristocracy of Spain, preferred living by themselves in the western and more fashionable parts of the city; and as neither them nor any of their families are sufficiently humble either to be engaged in trade or mix much with the lower ranks of people, their escape, during the epidemic of 1821, is nothing more surprising than that of the higher classes from the plague in London in 1666, the plague of Moscow in 1771, and many other instances before described. The west ends of London, Edinburgh and Glasgow, are like Barcelona in this respect ; they are all the most fashionable parts of these cities. What, therefore, Dr. O. observes of the yellow fever of Barcelona, begining in the eastern, and progressing towards the western parts of the city, accords exactly with what Dr. Willan says above, regarding the origin and mode of spreading of contagion in London.

Infected clothes are sold and conveyed in a thousand different ways in most large towns. At Constantinople, traffic in infected clothes is made a particular trade, and in Catholic countries, where masquerading is so much in vogue, the evils done in this way must be greater than with ourselves. We have no doubt that the great traffic in old clothes, carried on between Britain and Ireland, is one cause of the greater prevalence of typhus in the latter kingdom. As infected clothes and goods have no particular smell or mark by which they can be known, it is difficult to trace the spreading of contagion by such means.

Another cause of the difficulty of tracing contagion is the nonsusceptibility of certain individuals to its influence. If some persons receive or even wear infected clothes without experiencing any bad effects therefrom, a link in the chain of discovery is thus lost, and often leads to very erroneous conclusions concerning them.

A very interesting case of this kind is mentioned by Tully, which happened during the plague of Corfu. The complete success of the attacks made on plague by British bayonets, directed by the indefatigable generalship of His Excellency the late Sir Thomas Maitland, will long be remembered. This distinguished individual, alike regardless of all opinion and deaf to the scientific objections of medical men, proceeded at once to suppress pestilence, in the same way he did to bear down piracy,* and in both instances, the strong arm of power was equally successful and conspicuous. At this time, two Greek lovers who were betrothed to each other, happened unfortunately to be separated by one of the lines of circumvallation, part of which was bounded on one side by a river. The swain on this occasion, chanced to belong to the proscribed or infected district; the maiden, a beautiful Greek girl, to the healthy, and the house in which she lived along with her mother, was situated close to the bank of the river. For a time the two lovers could have no communication, excepting now and then holding a stolen conversation from the opposite banks of the stream, perhaps to enquire after each other's health. So long as the ardour of their love was thus restrained, all was well; but the young Greek on one occasion, threw a purse containing some money over the river, which was immediately picked up by the girl's mother, who, after keeping it some time, gave it to her daughter. The consequence of this act of kindness, was the death of the latter; she put the purse on receiving it into her bosom, and soon afterwards died of plague. The

* It was part of his policy to strike terror into the breasts of the Greek pirates, by hanging up the bodies of those who had been executed for piracy on some conspicuous height. Four men elevated in this way on the hills, in the island of Zante, got the name of Sir Thomas's Whist Party. We believe that many very interesting particulars might easily be picked up at Corfu concerning this plague. Sir Frederick Adam, the present governor, to whom we had the honour of being made known by the Hon. Sir Robert Spencer, kindly offered us every assistance in procuring information from the public records and elsewhere; but our time at Corfu was so uncertain and transitory, that we never had a good opportunity of performing the task, a thing we shall always regret.

mother, who was the first to receive the purse, remained
unhurt, although she kept it in her possession for some time.
A third cause of the difficulty of tracing contagion is, the
time it remains latent in the system before its effects become
manifest. Out of seventy-two cases of typhus fever, Doctor
Haygarth, found the latent period (allowing four days of
fever before the patient becomes infectious) was less than
ten days in only five, or probably in only three cases; that
it was less than seventeen days in only eleven or thirteen;
that it fell on some of the days between the seventeenth and
thirty-third day in forty-one, which is considerably more than
half the cases. It may be suspected, he adds, that the remaining sixteen patients who did not sicken, till a still longer
period had elapsed, might not be early and sufficiently exposed to the poison. " On the whole, it appears that the
latent period of infection varies from a few days to two
months."—*Letter*, p. 68.

The experience of Dr. Bancroft confirms the accuracy of
Dr. Haygarth's observations; for he found in ninety-nine
cases of orderlies and nurses, that attended the English army
on its arrival at Plymouth from Corunna, in 1809, that few
of them were attacked with fever earlier than the thirteenth
day, and in no instance later than the sixty-eighth day. Th
latent period of small-pox has been observed by many to be
from the fifth day to the sixteenth, seventeenth, and even the
twenty-third. In the casual or natural small-pox, the latent
period is a little longer.

Hydrophobia of all the contagions is the most uncertain
in its latent period; but as there are some well-authenticated
cases recorded of its occurring spontaneously or from causes
different from its effects, the exact time cannot always be accurately determined. Messrs. Magendi and Breschet have
succeeded in affecting a dog with rabies by inoculating him
with the saliva of a man under that disease. All doubts,
therefore, of its being a true contagion is now at an end.
Yet some cases are recorded by M. Rossi in the Mem. de

l'Academie de Turin, tom. 6th, which evidently demonstrate that animals previously healthy become capable, when enraged or irritated to a high degree, of communicating disease by their bite. The same fact appears to be decidedly established by Mr. James Gillman, for he records an instance where a dog that was chained in a yard without any kind of intercourse with diseased animals, had hydrophobia in its genuine form.—*Dissert. on the Bite of a Rabid Animal.* In the canine and feline species, about seven or eight days may be considered as a fair average of the shortest period in which the disease shows itself after the animal is bitten, and six or seven weeks the longest from the date of the bite. In the *human species* only a few days have in some instances elapsed previous to the symptoms showing themselves; but the most common time of their appearance is from twenty to forty days after the bite. Dr. Thomas thinks that there are no well-authenticated instances of the poison lying dormant longer than eleven or twelve months; and he, therefore, concludes that the instances mentioned by many authors, of several years having elapsed, have been cases of its spontaneous or equivocal production.

The following facts are stated by Dr. Bancroft regarding the typhus fever which prevailed among the British troops on their return from Corunna. Of thirty-five orderlies and nurses, who had returned from Spain, and therefore might have been previously exposed to contagion, it appeared that one was attacked on the first day after beginning to attend the sick; one on the 2nd, one on the 6th, two on the 7th, one on the 8th, one on the 9th, two on the 11th, one on the 14th, one on the 15th, one on the 16th, three on the 17th, one on the 18th, two on the 20th, one on the 21st, one on the 22nd, two on the 23d, two on the 24th, two on the 25th, one on the 26th, three on the 27th, one on the 28th, one on the 29th, one on the 38th, one on the 40th, and one on the 44th days. Of ninety-nine orderlies and nurses who *had not been out of England, nor* as far as was known *exposed to*

febrile contagion, it appears that one was attacked on the
13th day, one on the 14th, two on the 15th, one on the 16th,
four on the 18th, two on the 19th, three on the 20th, six on
the 21st, four on the 22d, four on the 23d, two on the 24th,
six on the 25th, four on the 26th, four on the 27th, eight on
the 28th, five on the 29th, three on the 30th, three on the
31st, two on the 33d, three on the 36th, four on the 37th,
one on the 38th, four on the 39th, one on the 40th, two on the
42d, three on the 44th, one on the 45th, five on the 47th, one
on the 48th, three on the 52d, two on the 54th, one on the
58th, one on the 60th, and one on the 68th days.   But these
returns, he adds, " were made up about the 20th April, and it
appears that some who had escaped till that time, were afterwards attacked, and therefore, though there may be reason to
conclude that febrile contagion does not remain inactive so
long after being received into the body as marsh miasmata,
I see none for believing that an interval *of five or six months*
may not sometimes elapse before the actual production of fever
by it, especially if the Summer should intervene previous to an
attack ; in which case the occurrence of fever would, I think,
almost always be postponed until the *following Winter,*
and often completely obviated ; and I cannot help strongly
suspecting that such a postponing of the disease happened to
some of the troops from Corunna in 1809.   It will be recollected that sickness prevailed to a very uncommon extent in
the army at home, during the early part of the preceding
year ; and though it did not consist exclusively of contagious
fever, that disease made a considerable part of it until it
became extinct at the approach of Summer.   It will also be
recollected that many of the regiments in whom this sickness
occurred, were, after its cessation, employed under Sir John
Moore and Sir David Baird in Spain, where typhus fever cannot exist in the Summer, and where, I believe, it never appears, even in Winter, *unless by an extraordinary introduction
of it.   Such an introduction took place* in this year by the
Spanish army under the Marquis de Romagna, which had

been removed from Holstein and Denmark (where typhus is a *frequent disease)* back to their own country in British transports."—Vide *On Yellow Fever, p.* 518.

Dr. Bancroft's ground for believing that the contagion of typhus fever may remain dormant in the system for the long period of five or six months, does not appear to be good, at least so far as he founds it *on an " extraordinary introduction of it"* into Spain by the return of the Marquis de Romagna's army to their own country; for, in the first place, such an extraordinary introduction could not be inferred merely from the circumstance of the Spanish army having come from Holstein and Denmark, where typhus is a *frequent disease ;* in the next, we do not recollect of having ever heard of a single case of typhus fever occurring on board of any of the British transports that conveyed them home. The transports containing the whole of that army were convoyed from the black rocks near Gottenburgh in Sweeden to Portsmouth, by his Majesty's ship Nassau, to which ship we then belonged. We had on board the Nassau a relation of the Marquis de Romagna, and several of the principal officers, besides the band of the regiment of Barcelona, and some of their wives. The general's aid-de-camp spoke good English, and with him we had much conversation during the passage, and as all reports concerning the state of the army on board the different transports were made to him, we had a good opportunity of knowing if such an extraordinary exportation of typhus contagion had really happened as Dr. Bancroft infers. Yet the fact is as we have stated it, though it is proper to add, we speak from recollection only. The Nassau's crew had a short time before suffered dreadfully from typhus fever (some account of which we have given before), so that this coincidence, had it happened, must have impressed the circumstance stronger on the mind. The weather at the time of the embarkation of the Spanish army in Sweeden was extremely hot, but, during the passage, it was surely sufficiently cool for the existence, in an active form, of typhus contagion.

The latent period is shorter in plague, which appears generally as early as the fourth or fifth day after exposure, and the
period of forty days, on which the law of quarantine has been
founded, will be found sufficient to secure the healthy from
the longest attack.   Yellow fever, as we shall afterwards see,
resembles plague in the shortness of the latent period.   But
in typhus, plague, and yellow fever, instances have occurred
of persons being taken unwell from the time of their first
exposure.   The late Professor Gregory of Edinburgh, mentioned a case of this kind in his lectures.   A young man
walking along the street, observed a heap of chaff, which he
struck with his foot in passing ; he instantly perceived a sick,
disagreeable smell to arise from it, which gave him a headach,
and afterwards typhus fever.   It was ascertained that the
chaff had been a short time before shaken out of a bed on
which a man had died of that disease.   Instances have fallen
within our own observation of persons being suddenly seized
with tremor on their first exposure, and remaining unwell till
the accession of fever.   In some of the cases, where a long
interval has occurred, it is likely that the clothes only were
infected, and that the individuals had not been exposed to a
sufficient dose of the poison ; in others, the system being pre-
occupied with other diseases, might have been the cause of
insusceptibility.   The difficulty of tracing contagion, must
be in proportion, in some measure, to the length of the interval between the exposure and the actual occurrence of disease.

A fourth cause of the difficulty of tracing it is, that the
action of the poison is liable to be suspended in other ways.
As before said, a hard frost may fix the subtle fluid to the
windows, in the same way it does other kinds of vapour or
gas; and here it will remain inactive till again set loose by
a thaw.   Hence, substances impregnated with the matter of
contagion may be rendered more dangerous by being exposed to heat, or the steam of warm water.   Variolous and
vaccine matter kept between two pieces of glass are breathed

on, or exposed to the steam of warm water, sometimes with this view; and women standing over a washtub containing infected clothes, have been seized with fever, while those persons who had handled them when they were cold received no injury. In like manner, the washing of the walls or wood of a house or ship with warm water, may probably become injurious to persons exposed to the operation. This is explained by the fact, that contagious effluvium is often sheltered in the pores of the wood and crevices of the walls : in these it is covered with a hardened crust or layer, formed by respirable and perspirable matters, and other emanations from persons and things which the apartment contained. This crust being once removed by the warm water, might not the contagious matter which was before fixed and protected, be exposed, softened, and let loose at the same time ? The matter of contagion while it remains in a gross or palpable form, might not be absorbed by the skin, but when volatilized by heat, will it not enter the lungs and stomach, especially in the close and ill-ventilated habitations of the poor in our own climate ? What we have stated above regarding the walls of houses, is rendered still more probable by the fact, that cases have occurred where every means of purification proved fruitless, till the rooms were painted, washed, or whitewashed. An instance was mentioned by the late Dr. Gregory, in his valuable lectures, where a person was infected with fever soon after taking possession of a house that had been empty for several months, and where it was ascertained, upon enquiry, that a family, some of whom had died of typhus, had been the last occupants.

" The last plague," says Dr. Parr (no mean authority), " that infected the town in which I write, arose from a traveller remarking to his companions, that in a former journey he had the plague in the room where they sat. ' In that corner,' said he, ' there was a cupboard where the bandages were kept; it is now plastered, but they are probably there still.'

He took the poker, broke down the plaster and found them. The disease was soon communicated and extensively fatal." —*Dictionary*, vol. i. p. 433.

It is proper to mention here some of the other modes in which the contagions are conveyed from place to place. Convalescents have frequently communicated them by mixing with healthy persons before they had sufficiently recovered or purified their persons and clothes. Many writers have observed, that convalescents from different diseases, are peculiarly prone to venereal pleasure. This fact was noticed by Dr. Rush, during the epidemic yellow fever of Philadelphia, in 1793; and Wilson, in his book on Febrile Diseases, Vol. II. p. 519, says, " So strong has the venereal appetite been in recoveries from plague, that it has often been known to counteract the endeavours of the magistrates in preventing the extension of contagion, as it tends of course to spread the distemper." According to Alderston, a mason who repaired the walls of a prison, where a prisoner had made his escape, was affected with contagious fever; and Doctor Haygarth, gives an instance of a cake of ginger-bread, that had been daubed with variolous matter, wrapt up in paper, and carried seventeen miles, infecting a child by whom it was eaten.

A street coach is another mode by which contagion is conveyed, without the least suspicion of those persons who become the sufferers. Coaches and chairs used to carry patients to hospitals, should be lined with wax-cloth instead of woollen-stuff or leather, as this does not retain or imbibe contagious effluvia, and may be washed as frequently as the outside or any part of the vehicle. Convalescents from febrile and other contagious diseases, it ought to be recollected, are frequently desired by their physicians to take a ride out in a coach, with a view to their complete recovery. When they first go out in this way, they are generally too imperfectly recovered to admit of the windows of a coach being kept open, so that the contagious effluvia emanating from their persons, stand a greater chance of being collected and imbibed, especially by woollen linings.

The very common practice (and one, too, more common amongst the working classes) of visiting persons ill of fevers, though it proceeds from good motives, likewise calls loudly for immediate attention. No sooner is it known that a person is taken seriously ill, than the chamber is filled with idle, and not unfrequently noisy visitants, a practice which not only increases the patient's danger, but multiplies in an incredible degree the seeds of disease. Dr. Ferriar says, " It may give us some idea of this danger to mention, that an elderly woman told me that she had fifteen children, all settled in the town, and all of whom had undergone the fever within two months."—Vol. iii. p. 53. Suppose this old woman had had two or more of her sons or daughters out at service, a thing by no means improbable, the seeds of contagion must have been conveyed to the families they served. Servants frequently ask leave of their masters or mistresses to go home to visit a sick relation ; and when this is obtained, the very first thing they do, is to act as nurse during the time they remain at home. Servants going at once from the large, clean and well-ventilated apartments of their masters, to the close and filthy abode of their relations, cannot but be doubly susceptible. However much, therefore, the practice may be commended in one point of view, it has undoubtedly been a source of incalculable mischief, not only to the servants themselves, but to the families whom they served. But besides this, there are in all great towns, numbers of old women who make a livelihood by keeping lodgings, or houses of call for servants ; and in order to enable themselves the better to do so, they add to their other occupation, that of sick nurse, both to rich and poor. These houses of call are filled every Sunday with servants from different places, who meet to discuss family politics and other matters, and very frequently they are asked to visit some of the numerous patients of their hostess. These, and the other circumstances before noticed, seem sufficient to explain the reason why, in all great contagious epidemics, servants have been observed to suffer in a greater proportion.

Beggars and vagrants of every description, may be looked upon as so many carriers of contagion, and the lodging-houses in which they assemble, as magazines for its preservation. It ought also to be borne in mind, that he who robs you of your goods, may rob you of your health at the same time, and by so doing, may actually do more harm by what he leaves behind than by what he takes away.

It has been supposed by some, that famine is a frequent cause of epidemics, and that it acts chiefly, if not wholly, by debilitating the constitutions of the poor; we are convinced this opinion is not well founded. During a scarcity of food at home, great numbers of people are forced to wander in search of a better supply; and as this increases begging and the intercourse above described, we surely cannot be surprised if contagious fevers are increased and multiplied at the same time. Now, as particular kinds of weather cause famine, and famine disease, the atmospheric influence has often been blamed also, and all the terrors of mystery called into play. Those would do less injury, did they not direct the minds of the people from the real sources of their maladies. During the epidemic typhus of 1815, 16, and 17, which was supposed to be occasioned chiefly by famine; the press teemed with practical treatises on the efficacy of blood-letting in that disease. Had debility from want of food been the only cause, the cure must have been very different.

Other animals convey contagion from place to place. Volney mentions the following:—" Il y a quelques années qu'un chat passait par les terrasses chez nos negocians à Caire et porta la peste a deux d'entre eux dont l'un mourait."

The flies in Egypt, we are convinced, frequently become inoculators of ophthalmia. The following instance fell under our own observation :—At Ægina, in Greece, there is a large seminary, where two or three hundred boys are taught the ancient and modern Greek tongues, and other branches of education. This school is divided into several class-rooms, which are large, high in the roof, and well aired and lighted. They likewise communicate with each other by doors in the inside, so that free communication between the different classes, can either be given or withheld as occasion might require. The building is divided into wings, and there is a large square and play-ground in the centre. At the time we visited the place, which was in August, 1829, we found the true Egyptian ophthalmia, committing its direful ravages amongst the pupils; almost every one had either gone through the disease, or was suffering severely from it. On entering the square along with another officer, the poor little fellows surrounded us in scores, and pointing to their eyes, eagerly asked for relief. Upon enquiry, we were told that some of the boys who had been taken from the Morea to Egypt, by Ibram Pacha, had imported the disease on their return. Our impression was, that the malady might have been at first easily kept from spreading in the school, by cutting off the communication between the different classes and parts of the building, till we recollected, that the flies, which swarmed in every apartment and in every place, must have rendered all attempts of this kind abortive; on en-quiry, we found our second thought to be the most correct.

Several of the great epidemics on record, either derived their origin from smuggling, or smugglers were the first victims. The last plague of Malta, the yellow fever of Cadiz in 1800, and that of Malaga of 1803, are instances. In the last case, the dead body of a man was not only brought on shore, but actually smuggled into a grave in a church-yard; but to give a correct notion of the innumerable modes in which disease might easily be introduced into a country by such means, would be to write a treatise on illicit trade, and the comparative merits of revenue laws. Although the prac-tice of smuggling is daily and nightly carried on almost in every country where it can be made the means of gain, yet, strange to say, the difficulty of ascertaining the importation of a disease into a place in this way, by direct evidence, has been laid hold of by the non-contagionists, and applied as a kind of splint to prop up their lame and broken theory; and in order to make their splint apply better and sit somewhat more easily, they soften down the stiff unbending pieces with the oath of the smugglers themselves, and finish their clumsy operation by wrapping up the whole in mystery.

To conclude our observations on the mode of spreading, " religious functions, charitable offices, official duties, public spectacles and amusements, multiply the sources of infection, and may carry contagion from the cottage to the palace."*

There are no facts in the history of contagion better ascertained or more generally admitted, than that very few susceptible persons will escape an attack of a contagious disease when exposed to a concentrated dose of the poison in close and badly ventilated apartments; on the other hand, few will suffer from its influence in large airy and clean places : in fact, the number of individuals attacked in different places, will be found to correspond very much with their circumstances in these respects. In March, 1793, a fever, attended with alarming symptoms, was brought from the jail among the inhabitants of a narrow lane, near the White Cross (Newcastle); it appeared as follows :—In a family occupying a *small room* and a *closet, seven* persons were infected; in another house, the family occupying *two rooms, three* were infected; in a third house, the family occupying *two rooms, one* person was infected; and in a fourth house, the family occupying *two rooms, two* were infected. This fever was taken to Gateshead nearly about the same time; also, in Wall Knoll; in another house, the family occupying *two rooms,* one of which was *under ground, seven* persons were infected; in a sixth house, the family occupying *one room, two* were

---

* See Stanger, p. 20.

infected. In a lane at Quarry Side, a similar fever appeared in a house, the family occupying *one* room, *seven* persons were infected. The disease from this house was carried to Sandgate and to Castle Garth about the same time; in a house, the family occupying *one* room, containing two beds, *six* persons were infected; in the same house, another family occupying a different room, *three* persons were infected; in another family, occupying a third room in the same house, *five* were infected; in a fourth room of the same house, *one*, making in all *fifteen persons in a single house.*

According to Haygarth, one in twenty-three or thirty-three will escape infection on exposure to the contagion of typhus fever, if exposed a sufficient length of time in filthy, close and ill-ventilated apartments; and the same author gives instances of seventeen and eighteen persons being infected in a single family; and he adds, " though an induction from facts never amounts to a demonstrative proof, yet, the further it is carried, it approaches the nearer towards a complete discovery of the laws of Nature."—Vide *Letter to Dr. Perceval,* p. 32.

Much has been said about this want of what is called direct proof, and many very erroneous conclusions have been drawn from it; but if we apply the doctrine of chances to the facts we have brought forward, what would be the result ? I proposed, says Dr. Stokes, the following problems to a friend, particularly acquainted with this species of computation. 1st. An epidemic prevails so severe that *one* of *seven* sickens : a family of *twelve* is selected in a particular district before the epidemic has visited it : What is the chance that *eleven* out of this family should take the disease, supposing the sickness of one of the family does not promote the sickness of another, and supposing the family not unusually liable to disease ? The answer is, that the probability against the event is nearly 189,600,000 to 1, *if the population amount to* 7,000. 2nd. The same conditions being assumed, what is the chance that, *in any family* of twelve, within the district, eleven will sicken? Answer; it is above 300,000 to 1, that no family of twelve will have eleven sick.—Vide *Stokes on Contagion*, pp. 23-24. Let us apply the same principles to the epidemic cholera now prevailing in Sunderland, where six in one family were attacked, five of whom died. Let us suppose that Sunderland contains seven thousand inhabitants, and that one thousand out of the seven had been attacked with the disease, the chance that six, which in the Sunderland case we believe was the whole number the family contained, sicken in one family, is 117,649 to 1 against the event.* But the population of Sunderland being more than twice this number, and those actually affected only 400, the probabilities against it were infinitely greater.

Dr. Ferriar, vol. ii. p. 195, states, "that a house in a very confined situation had been infected during several years in three of the rooms, and at one time, when the whole family was ill, four persons died from want of the common offices of a nurse. During all this time, an elderly couple who lodged in the fourth room, separated from the infected only by the narrow staircase of the house, preserved themselves from disorder, merely by avoiding all communication with the rest of the family."—*Medical Histories*.

Some years ago we visited a farmer's family in the country, which consisted of six persons, including the father and mother, and nine individuals, including three servants : the whole number went through typhus fever one after the other, at a time when not a single case of that disease was to be found in the immediate neighbourhood. Many of the neighbours visited this family daily at the time of their illness, but as their visits were short, and the sick apartments pretty well ventilated, none of them took the fever.

The Rev. Joseph Townsend, wrote Dr. Haygarth thus :—
" When I had my putrid fever, I took it from my gardener,

---

* This computation was made by our friend E. P. Fordham, Esq. civil engineer, on whose accuracy the public may depend.

and he received it from a poor cottage. My room was well ventilated, and no one caught it from me. Mr. Stephens took the infection from a poor patient, but no one received it from him; both houses were well ventilated. In the year 1787, out of two hundred poor families, sixty-three poor people died of typhus, but no other farmer or principal tradesman had this fever. When one family died of it, another succeeded to their cottage, and the new comers caught the fever."

The fever which broke out at the Old Baily Sessions in 1750, and which attacked the Lord Mayor, several of the Judges, the Under-Sheriff, and many of the Middlesex Jury, besides others, raged for about six weeks, but did not spread from the individuals who were exposed in court. Had its victims been persons in a humble rank of life, and of course obliged to inhabit close and ill-ventilated apartments, the result in all probability would have been very different.

Having now laid before the reader, the principal facts at present known concerning marsh and morbid poisons, with a view to their prevention and removal, and explained the different phenomena connected with the rise, progress, and decline of endemic, epidemic, and contagious diseases on known principles, it is necessary, before finishing this part of the work, to make a few general observations. In grappling with a subject so extensive and difficult, we thought it best to bring the facts to bear closely on the most disputed points, with a view of rendering them as near demonstrative evidence as the nature of the subject would admit. Any one who will take time calmly and dispassionately to consider these facts and the arguments founded upon them, must, we think, come to the conclusion, that known principles are adequate to explain most, if not all the mysteries that have continued so long to obscure the causes of marsh and contagious diseases.

As the effects of marsh and morbid poisons have generally been confounded, and the influence of the atmosphere on these causes of disease and on the diseases themselves, has frequently been misunderstood, it has been our endeavour to ascertain what share each of these powerful agents has in producing that frightful catalogue of human ills that has usually been attributed to their single or joint operation. The best way of doing this seems to be, first to ascertain all the known properties of the three agents separately; for while every writer who has a favourite theory to support continues to ascribe to the atmosphere, to marsh poison and to contagion, whatever property he pleases, or that best suits his views, it is impossible to arrive at anything like fixed principles. We have therefore considered very fully these important and extensive causes of disease in three separate dissertations ; as in this way the reader will be better able to detect us, if in any thing we have swerved from the principles we have laid down. The present state of knowledge regarding them having been once ascertained and their individual or respective properties fixed, our next endeavour was to find out the influence each has upon the other. In doing this we have not been guided by prejudice, having no favourite hypothesis to support, nor new doctrine to bring forward. We agree with Dr. Johnson, in thinking that " what is known is rejected, because it is not sufficiently considered that men more frequently require to be *reminded* than *informed*." All that is wanted to secure us against contagious diseases is, to take a due advantage of the knowledge we already possess. Unfortunately the mode in which they are to be prevented interferes with private interests, a circumstance which serves partly to account for a doctrine frequently promulgated, namely, that nothing is known regarding the properties of contagion. The mischievous tendency of such a doctrine need scarcely be pointed out, as a belief in it can never lead to any useful practical result. " That which in speculation stands for the cause, is what in practice stands for the rule ;" but " from torpid despondency can come no advantage, it is the frost of the soul which binds up all its powers and congeals life in perpetual sterility. He that has no hopes of success will make no attempt, and where nothing is attempted nothing can be done."

We wish particularly to draw the public attention to the great importance of *Statistical Medicine*, a branch of science which has been much neglected. As well might the physician try to account for the corrupted state of the fluids of the human body without a knowledge of the diet and regimen of his patient, as to attempt an explanation of the different phenomena connected with the history of epidemical diseases without a constant reference to the actions of men and the state and condition of society. We are well aware that some, who possess a peculiar taste for the abstract and sublime, will accuse us of having chosen a vulgar occupation, and also, of giving much trite and common-place matter. As these philosophers not unfrequently proceed to build a structure without even a foundation, so they expect others to raise one without the props and small stones which are necessary to support the larger. The question of contagion or non-contagion is one which involves too many serious considerations to be made the subject of loose or unguarded speculation at any time; but at present, it is undoubtedly one of the most important that can possibly engage the attention of mankind. The pomp of power, the aggrandizement of states, and the forwarding of party views and interests, may indeed assume a more inviting and promising aspect; but even questions as to these must sink into insignificance, when compared with one which so deeply interests the whole human race—when pestilence spreads disease and death around, all calculations on human greatness must be poor indeed.

It may be thought odd, that we have said so little about Cholera, but this is not a book written on any particular disease. It has been our object to teach general principles rather than to lay down insulated rules. The latter are

seldom observed where the principles on which they are
founded remain unknown; and any one who will take the
trouble of examining what we have said of contagion in
general, will be able to judge how far cholera is regulated by
the same laws. So long as principles are confined to works
purely medical, they have little chance of being seen by the
general reader, or, if at all noticed by him, they are apt to
be confounded or obscured, either by the language in which
they are almost always wrapt up, or the speculative opinions
with which they are but too frequently accompanied. The
prevention of disease depends more on the public in general,
than on the medical portion of the community. It is therefore a matter of the utmost importance that they should be
made acquainted with the principal facts known concerning
atmospheric influence, marsh miasmata and contagion, as
without this, they are sure to fall a prey to the sophistry of
the learned, the machinations of the interested, or the prejudices of the ignorant.

Had the people of Malta been aware of the narrow sphere
of contagion in 1830, those of Moscow of the power of frost
in suspending the contagion of plague in 1720, and had the
government of Gibraltar acted at once on the principles of
contagion in 1804, instead of pinning their faith to a mere
opinion, countless thousands of human beings might have easily
been saved from destruction.

Although the bad effects of a wrong opinion of contagion are seldom, if ever, confined to those who embrace it,
but prove equally destructive to others; yet we know no
subject on which speculation is oftener indulged or exercised,
and certainly none in which mankind have profited so little
by past experience. Every one who has heard the terms
contagion and infection and believes he understands their
true signification, seems to think himself justified in promul-
gating his opinion. The tyro in medicine who has seen a
few cases of cow-pox or measles, the quack who owes his
reputation to the ignorance of his patients, and the parent

who has observed disease chiefly within the circle of his own family, frequently boast of having made up their minds on the subject; and it will generally be observed, that each individual becomes stubborn or otherwise in proportion to his ignorance. We cannot, therefore, too strongly warn the public of the danger of listening to the crude and flimsy effusions of the newspaper press, on the subject of cholera and contagion in general. Many of these productions have evidently been written by men of some talent, but who think it a mark of greater wisdom to dissent from the opinions of the better-informed and more experienced. According to them, age is imbecility, caution is cowardice, wisdom is folly, and knowledge any thing but power.

Two years ago we gave it as our opinion, that the Asiatic Cholera is contagious, and that it would ultimately reach this country; we see no reason to alter this opinion. Much has been said about contingent contagion; what contagion does not depend upon contingencies. Throughout the whole of this dissertation, therefore, it has been our particular study to point out the necessity of attending to these very contingencies or concurrences of circumstances, before we can account either for the generation of a contagion or for its after-spreading. Cholera is an exotic plant, and may not be able to spread out its roots and branches so easily in Britain, as it does on its native soil. That imperfect and spurious forms of the disease may be more frequent with us, and that such forms of the malady are not contagious, are things not to be wondered at by any one who carefully peruses the foregoing sheets; but had we no other facts to prove its contagion than those furnished by the history of its ravages in Sunderland, these would warrant the wise precautionary measures adopted by Government.

An agent floating in the atmosphere of a place, is just as likely to affect one individual living in it as another, supposing that all are equally susceptible of its influence, for we know of no way by which that atmosphere can be breathed by one person and avoided by another. Let us suppose that the town of Sunderland and its immediate neighbourhood contains 15,000 inhabitants, which we believe is nearly its population, and that five hundred persons have been attacked with cholera, then one person in thirty would be the proportion of sick on the atmospheric theory ; but if one individual out of a family containing six persons was seized, then it would have five times its proportion of sick ; so that even in this case the balance would be in favour of contagion. What then must be our conclusions, if *six*, *the whole number the family contained*, be attacked with the disease, and *five* out of the *six* die, the chance against such an event is *some hundreds of thousands to one*.

Again, the cholera of Sunderland has already attacked more than four hundred persons, including the mild cases, and it has proved fatal to more than one in three and a half. Yet we are told by some that it is only a British disease, and one derived from the atmosphere. We have before given the annual number of deaths in London from bowel-complaints, (which includes cholic, flux, gripes, &c.) taken from an average of ten years, at the beginning, middle, and end of the eighteenth century, when the whole deaths were about 21,000. By this document, viz. the bills of mortality, it appears that 1,100 died of these complaints in one year at the beginning, 135 at the middle, and only twenty at the end of that century ; so that out of a population of about 600,000, only twenty persons, or one in thirty thousand, die of *every thing in the shape of bowel-complaint in a whole year* in London; whereas, in Sunderland, out of a population of 15,000, one hundred persons die, or 1 in 150, *of one single form* of disease in *a few weeks*, and that too in a mild season, and in an age when the mode of living is so much improved. Query—If a British disease kills only twenty persons out of *six hundred thousand in one year*, what is the probability that a malady which kills *five out of six persons* in a family in *a few weeks*, is also a British disease ?

Lastly, this aerial vision attacks 400 persons in a population of 15,000, and is confined to *one small spot only* of the
British dominions at home, where it was never before heard
of. From this fact two questions arise : the first is—What
is the probability that 400 persons be attacked with a British
atmospheric disease out of 15,000 persons, *at a time when
the whole population of England, Ireland, and Scotland,
remains in its usual healthy state ?* The other is—What is
the chance that such an occurrence should take place in the
latter end of the year 1831, when the whole British dominions at home have remained free from a similar mortality
during the whole period of well-authenticated history ? Those
who are acquainted with political arithmetic and the doctrine
of chances, may answer these important questions. The
numbers of course have been coarsely stated, but the principle is sufficiently plain. We have no doubt but many
persons will be found, whose powers of deglutition are such
as to get over these difficulties without much hesitation ; but,
let these recollect, that the mortality in London was not
taken from one year, twenty deaths was the annual mortality
on an average of ten years. Perhaps no country in Europe
offers greater facility, in some respects, to the spreading of
pestilence than Britain ; for, although some possess a more
dense and less enlightened population, yet in no other is
there the same degree of intercourse and communication
between persons and goods. Such is the facility and rapidity
of travelling, that the most distant parts of this kingdom
may be said to approximate each other. A great proportion
of our population depends upon intercourse for their subsistence. The staple commodities of our trade are woollen
and cotton goods, which are of all other substances the best
adapted for entertaining and conveying contagion. A foreign
disease which has been introduced into the island by trade,
is more likely to maintain its connexion with commercial
transactions, than one propagated in the usual way by domestic intercourse. The people are unaccustomed to com-

mercial restrictions. We have no system of medical police or laws which can sanction their perfect adoption; the public are ignorant, or at least unpractised in the means of prevention. Our medical men are unacquainted with cholera, and their minds are unsettled as to its nature; ignorant and uneducated persons are allowed to practise medicine; the newspaper press to circulate injurious medical opinions, &c. &c. We do not presume to find fault with this state of things in ordinary times; we only mention them as circumstances which favour the spreading of contagion. While they remain the same, the measures of Government will not prove effectual, any more than they will be in preventing intercourse and communication; a want of confidence in the means of prevention will follow, the prejudices of the public will be increased, and the disease in all probability will become general. The stagnation of trade, the general distress and famine, the loss to the revenue, the expence of quarantine hospital and other establishments, the increase of poor-rates and burdens of the people, and the temptation to robbery, and other crimes that will undoubtedly attend this unhappy result, it is frightful to contemplate. The question therefore naturally suggests itself, whether it is better to submit to partial privations, in order to check the progress of the disease at first, or run the risks just mentioned? If the small portion of the community amongst whom the disease is still confined, suffer for the larger, their pecuniary losses may be made up to them; but if the larger portion suffer for the smaller, by what means could the loss to the nation be compensated? We do not pretend to be sufficiently acquainted with the spirit of our laws to be able to recommend the adoption of any particular system of prevention; but speaking medically, that system is the best which most prevents intercourse between infected and healthy places, which strikes at the root of the evil, by promoting the cleanliness and increasing the comforts of the poor. "What can so strongly demand the attention of the

Legislature, as the health and strength of the great mass of the people: objects to be attained by measures which are also conducive to private happiness and virtue, to public order and economy, and to national wealth and power.''

Let us unite, therefore, in endeavouring to avert, or at least to lessen, the evil of this awful visitation. Let the ignorant and prejudiced be informed, the selfish and interested abate their desire of gain; let the pedant pause before he promulgates his opinions, the libertine cease to boast of his freedom; let the politician dismiss from his heart the rancour of party spirit, the dogmatist learn from past experience; let the indolent rouse from their slumbers, and the rash become acquainted with danger; let all these read the history of cholera.

This scourge of supposed atmospheric origin, has travelled in a *slow and gradual manner* over a great portion of the civilized world, keeping pace not with the winds, but making its journeys at the rate of travelling in the countries it visits. No climate, season, or soil, can retard its progress: it rages in hot, in cold, and in temperate regions; in high winds and in calm weather, in great droughts and in torrents of rain, in mountainous districts and in level plains, in countries well-cultivated, and in those in a barren or desert state; on places rich in soil and places having no soil; it has travelled over seas and over rivers, in the face of a gale of wind or with the wind; it is regardless of the laws which regulate caloric, magnetism, or the electric fluid: in short, it mocks at repulsion, holds out its finger at chemical attraction, and stalks in terrible array over every species of matter; and what is the reason of all this? The answer cannot be mistaken—it is nursed in the lap of society, and conveyed from place to place by intercourse and communication.

END OF THE FIFTH DISSERTATION.

Printed by G. HAYDEN, Little College Street, Westminster.

INDEX.

Milton Keynes UK
Ingram Content Group UK Ltd.
UKHW041521181024
449640UK00009B/125